Serious Muscle Enhancement

18 week

Muscle-building Course

Serious Muscle Enhancement 18 week
Muscle building Course

By

Birch Tree Publishing
Published by Birch Tree Publishing

The Serious Muscle Enhancement Manual was designed to showcase my gains with Stress Methods that explain various muscle-stimulating techniques in great detail. It essentially kick-started the Beyond muscle-building stress methods—and the gains of muscle-sculpting trainees all over the world.

Tables of Contents

INTRODUCTION

Imagine packing on solid ripped pounds of muscle on your physique in a matter of a few weeks. Even a few pounds of sculpted muscle will make a massive difference on your frame.
That amount of muscle distributed on a trainee's frame will turn the smallest stick figure into an amazing physical marvel. Even10 pounds would put the trainee in the superman category. Unfortunately, it takes most trainees some time to gain favorable muscle. However, I am often asked why does the growth process take forever most times? The reason-most trainees do not eat enough which will obstruct the muscle-building process along with workouts that are simply a waste of time.

Those two problems translate into little, and most times zero, muscle growth for extended periods. This muscle-sculpting plan will help you avoid those haphazard practices with a sound program that will push your physique to new levels in record time, as it did for me.
 My 15-pounds-of-muscle gain in 12 weeks happened in 1993. It was the result of an experiment with a size-building method and program that I constructed. I have been researching training and eating strategies for building muscle for more than 30 years, which is why I am motivated by my experiments.

The program is a simple one, so please follow it if you want to achieve the best muscle and strength gains possible. However, I must mention that maximum motivation is a must so please give every rep and set your all. Convince yourself that you're going to pack on as much sculpted lean muscle as possible with the training, and as night follows day, you will have just that.

I will continue to research muscle growth, refining the key components of muscle growth that originally spurred the development of a number of effective stress methods and techniques. The plan will be to amplify the key muscle-building components—which I will do , as I've packed on more pounds of ripped muscle year after year with each and every experiment So, give the muscle-enhancing-program your best shot, and you will be guaranteed a physical transformation—in only 18 short weeks—that will literally astound your friends and family.

--Marlon Birch--

CHAPTER 1
THE BEGINNING TO MUSCULAR GROWTH ENHANCEMENT

Like most young men who start any form of exercise, I had dreams of being big and powerfully muscular, that made people stare when I walked down the street. However, my biggest dream was competing in bodybuilding shows. Charles Atlas and Steve Reeves were a massive influence, and their physiques represented what I was striving for—but I understood that I would never build an Arnold type physique, but kept going regardless due to my quest for strength.

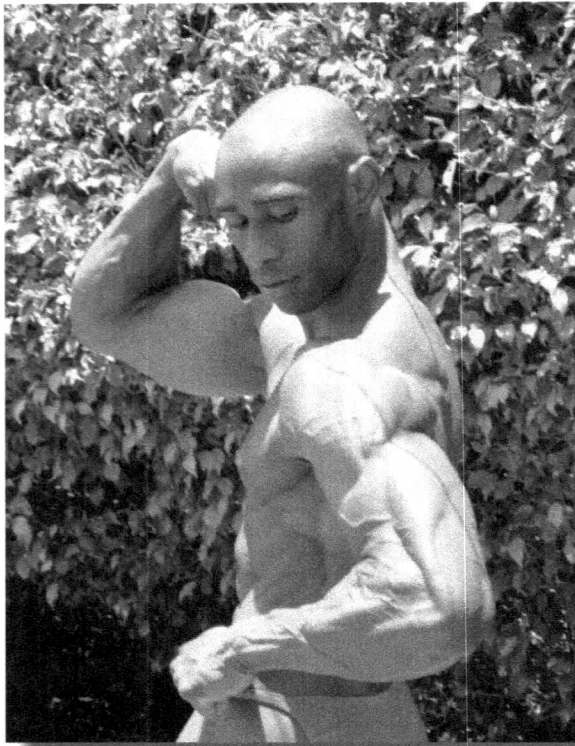

After a few years I progressed to a respectable level of muscle-size, my dream got closer and closer, which got me more motivated to see where I would end up with it all.

Later years I entered my first contest—with lots of coaxing from the guys I worked with. I knew I needed much more muscle size to make an impressive mark, but I entered anyway, primarily to prove to myself that I can do this.

The guys kept telling me I couldn't compete successfully without lifting weights and the self-resistance I am doing. They stated, I will get cut and not much bigger.

Their words echoed throughout my mind and I stated, look at the results I have achieved already! So, instead of an argument I used what they said to fuel my intensity. Which made me stronger and I believed that I could do it without weights.

While I did make an impressive showing at my first contest, the real size I was seeking did not stand fast. I wasn't BIG enough one judge said. However, it did not deter my interest in training for it was still strong, another judge told me he liked my shape and I am balanced. That got me even more motivated and excited! I took to the books and trained hard, ate well and consistently focused on doing my best on each rep. The results was documented and all the nay-sayers were very shocked by the results I got from my various programs. Which is what I needed to keep moving forward.

CHAPTER 1

My bodypart measurements and strength increases were quite serious. As the title states Serious Muscle Enhancement. Now, unbelievable I know —and I did this with a sensible self resistance training program, along with combined science, and a consistent eating schedule. However, these gains were miraculous to say the least. Adding new muscle that quickly felt awesome! I want to pass on my experience and stress methods I made the second time around with the Muscle Enhancement program—in hopes that you, too, can make rapid progress in size, conditioning and power. It was an amazing, muscle-building experience—and I finally got the physique I was after. Maybe you'll be able to build as much as 20 plus pounds of muscle in18 weeks! For most trainees have superior genetics, far greater than mine. So give it a serious go.

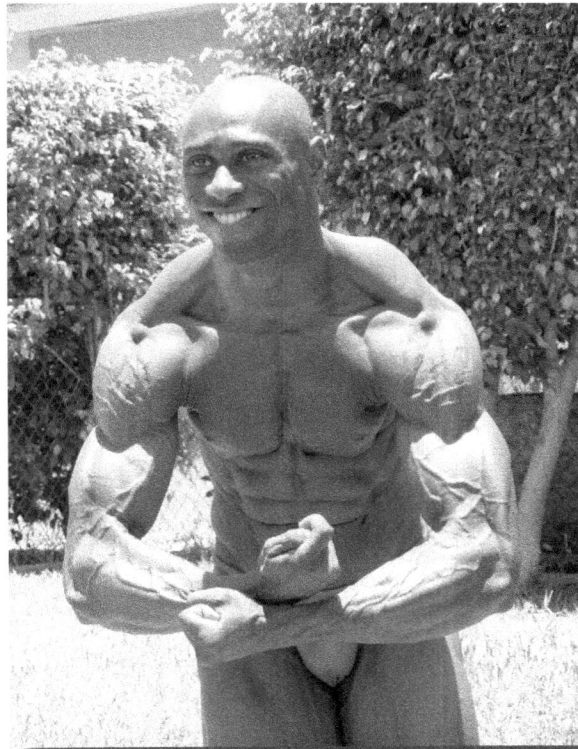

Above after perfecting the Muscle Enhancement stress methods at 1.4% bodyfat

CHAPTER 1

Before beginning this program do not do any exercise for at least ten days—no arguments. After the rest you can move on to the high-intensity regimen outlined in this book. However, please note: If you haven't been exercising for a few months and you need to get back into exercise or you are a complete beginner, I recommend you start with The Beyond Self Resistance Mini course Workout 1. After that start up regimen, you can move to Phase 1 of this Serious Muscle Enhancement program followed by the Beyond Self Resistance BodyBuilding Manual.

As you will see in the next chapter, the first three weeks of the Muscle Enhancement program is a basic six-days-per-week routine. Attack this with full force! What happened is that I got much bigger than I'd ever been, so I gained over 12 pounds of new muscle on the Muscle Enhancement program—and more on a second go of the system.

As you will notice, the overall training scheme in the Serious Muscle Enhancement program is broken down into a few-high-intensity training phases, the reason for the shorter-intensity 3 week phases is simple—the body adapts within a 4-6 week cycle. So to prevent full adaptation there is a back off so the body can handle more stress. When your body encounters a repeated form of stress like high-intensity strength resistance training, it will go through three levels of adaptation:

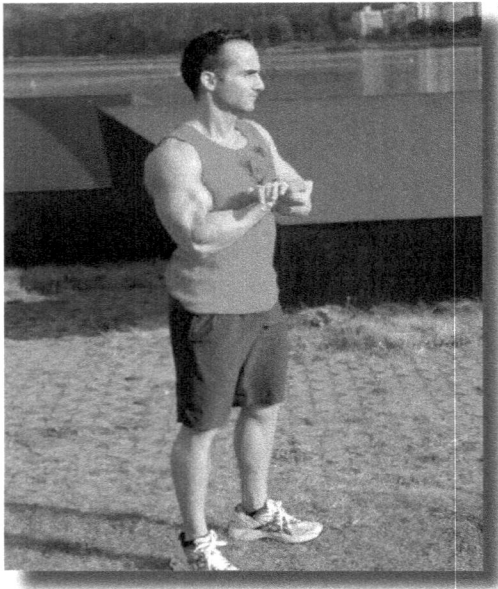

1) Adjustment Phase.
   During the first week of training your body begin by adjusting and will compensate from the new irritation by getting slightly weaker due to new stress.

2) Adaptation Phase.
   During the first two-three weeks your body actually adapts to the training irritation by getting leaner and stronger.

3) Hyper-Growth Phase. As the body continues to grow and get stronger due to new stimuli, no plateau takes place, and no regression will occur. By shifting into a different training module after three weeks of high-intensity training, you avoid adaptation entirely.

 In other words, you go from adjustment to adaptation, back to adjustment and then to adaptation again—you get continuous muscle-enhancing stimulation, in a 18-week period.

CHAPTER 1

Let's check out the program...

Phase One
Day One

Decline pushups
Liederman press
Crossed feet squats
Resisted leg extensions
Leg curls
Resisted leg extensions
Leg curls
Resisted pulldowns
Three chair dips
Across the body rows
Decline pushups (elbows out)
Resisted shoulder press
Resisted upright rows

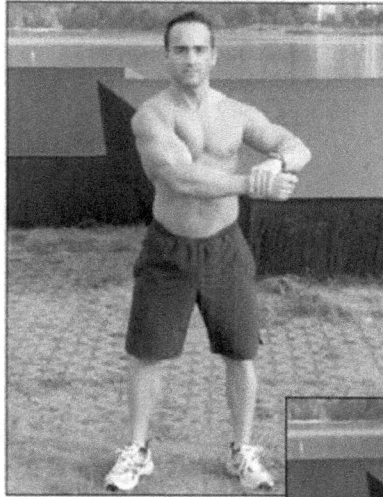

Day Two
Thigh rows
Standing calve raises
Reverse crunches
Across the body rows
Resisted forward tricep press
Tricep pressdown
Bicep curl palm up
Reverse curls
Palm up wrist curls

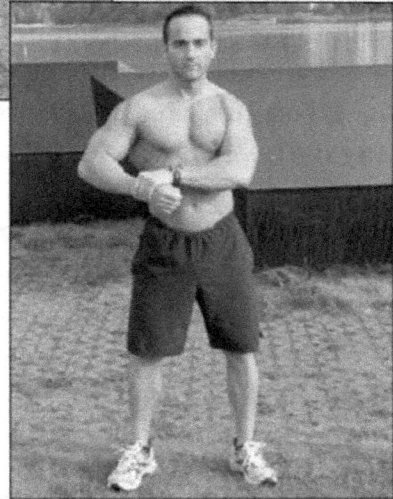

CHAPTER 1

Day Three

Crossed feet squats
Resisted leg extensions
Resisted leg curls
Standing calve raises
Decline pushups
Liederman press
Resisted pulldown
Across the body rows
Decline pushups (elbows out)
Resisted shoulder press
Resisted upright rows

Perform all reps at 10-15, sets 3-4. This is a 6 day a week training protocol.

What is the the key to the exercise plan?
It is a full-range muscle-building protocol that can help you build lean muscle quickly.
It's packed as much as 12 plus pounds of muscle onto my frame in as little as 12 weeks.

My various friends all over the world have found it to be a straight-forward, scientific training approach that's based on muscle function, and it's extremely efficient (no wasted effort, which means efficient workouts!). Once you light the fuse, you will get more strength and muscular growth bang for your biceps than you have ever experienced before—once you don't abuse the stress methods.

My system shows you how to choose exercises that train each muscle through its entire range of motion, or ROM, to coax extraordinary fiber recruitment at every workout. That means faster, more complete muscle development from fewer sets...........

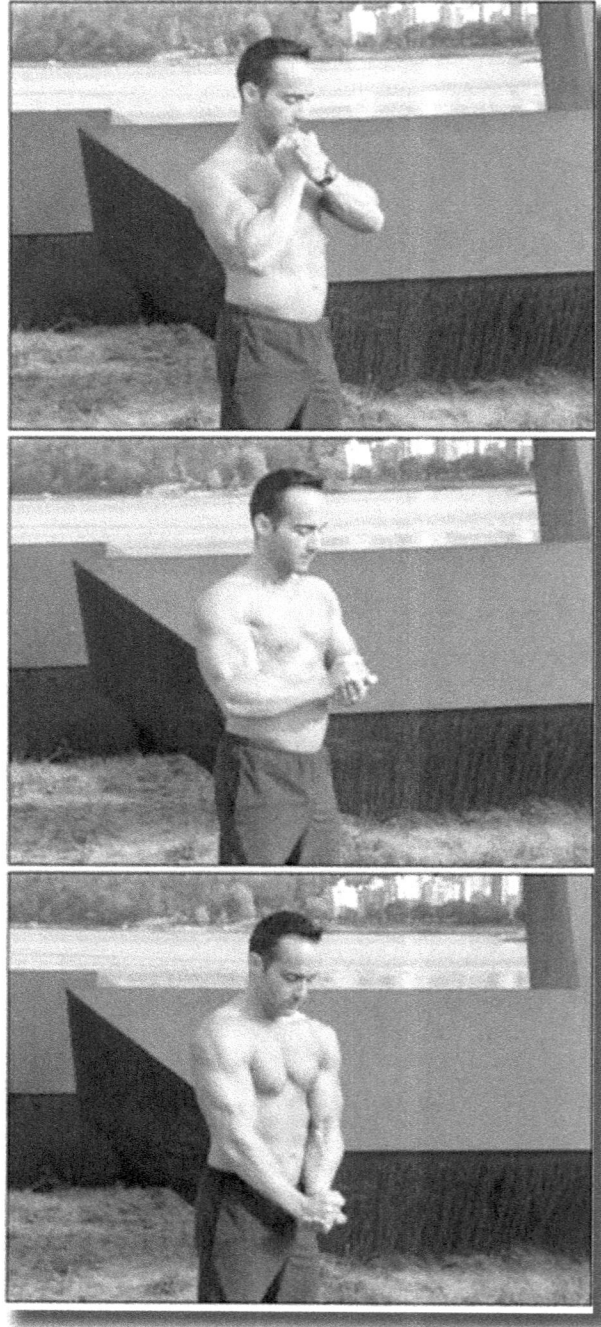

CHAPTER 1

The Muscle Enhancement Program allows you to work a muscle's full arc of flexion—which build muscle and strength fast! You'll feel it happening! Achieving full range for a muscle may take one, two or three exercises (sometimes one exercise can cover two arcs of flexion), but it never takes more than three to get the job done. That complete multi-angular attack develops fuller muscles by triggering more fibers to fire—which may startle you the first time you try it if you're new to self resistance full range protocol.

In fact, many self resistance trainees express their surprise, even shock, after putting it to the test, commenting that they thought their skin might tear because the influx of blood while performing the workouts. That's a direct result of the extreme muscle coaxing recruitment you get when you train a target muscle with effiencientcy of effort. An immediate force production via a full-blown pump. The target muscles get so much stimulation that there's a massive blood flow to the area after only a few sets. This conditioning is what the trainee should strive for— The pump is a signal that the muscle has been stressed enough to produce muscle-building-stimulation, it helps create an environment in which more of the fibers can be stimulated.

By stretching the fascia sheetings, the muscle-fiber encasements, that can restrict growth if it is left to remain tight. The key to the effectiveness is continuous tension, no rest during the set, which blocks blood flow to the muscle. That occlusion is a powerful anabolic stimulus and also produces a potent anabolic jolt after then heightened fiber activation created by a pre-stretch-position exercise. Once you understand the concept, you can see why my program works and why it creates a skin-stretching pump in only a few sets. You totally stimulate the muscle fibers by triggering the stretch reflex in a routine that trains each bodypart then forces the muscle to contract forcefully.

VOLUME VS INTENSITY:
HOW TO ACHIEVE MAXIMUM LEAN MUSCLE GROWTH

Which is more important for muscle growth, volume (the amount of work done in a workout) or intensity (the effort of each set)? Alot of trainees draw the line in the sand and think you need to be on one side or the other. Truthfully, there's more than one way to look at this. If your muscles are exposed to intensity levels for the same amount of time over and over, they will not grow. Your workouts must change to coax your body to adapt and change—either workouts become more intense or you increase the volume (more sets, and reps).

The best way to irritate the muscles is to opted for the volume method, along with stress methods tacked on but, never train to failure, intensity should be in the medium range. A trainee can flirter with training to muscular exhaustion on a few sets, usually after three to four subfailure (medium-intensity) sets—but training too intensely for long periods would lead to burnout and regression, so backing off frequently is needed.

CHAPTER 1

If a trainee prefer workouts with brutal intensity. (which, I do not recommend). Every work set taken to complete exhaustion with massive force and beyond with only a few sets per bodypart; this can lead to tendon damage over time. So which way should the trainee train? In an ideal situation you would use both—a three-week phase of volume training followed by a week of short subfailure supercompensation workouts followed by another three-week phase of high-intensity style training followed by another week of subfailure supercompensation training and so on.

Most times I train at night, so I lean toward volume intensity-style workouts; however, once stress methods are applied with slight volume increases trigger new muscle gains, as does heightened intensity. Frequent change equals bigger muscle coaxing gains. Keep that in mind as you move into specific muscle-coaxing-tactics for each muscle position. Here's the Muscle Coaxing masterplan, along with a brief review of each of those positions of flexion.

MUSCLE-TEAM-WORK: Force Generation
PRE-STRETCH POSITION: Pre-Stretch Generation
CONTRACTION POSITION: Continuous Tension/Occlusion Output

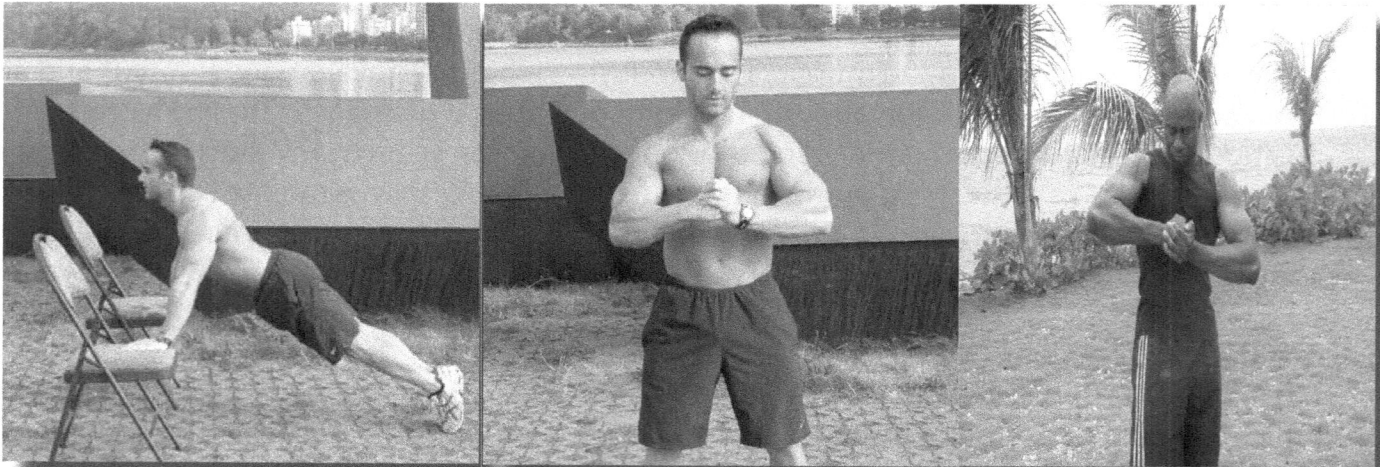

MUSCLE-TEAM-WORK: Stimulates the bulk of the muscle fibers with muscle teamwork. When a number of muscles work together—such as the chest, triceps and shoulders during decline pushups—the target (chest) is more effectively stimulated with being pre-stretched and muscular overload. The human muscle structures are designed to work in tandem for maximum power, so these movements generate maximum muscular generation. Example: one legged squats, pushups, and thigh rows.

CHAPTER 1

PRE-STRETCH: Pre-Stretch: Here you put the target muscle in its ultimate elongated, or stretched, state under resistance. The stretch triggers the stretch reflex, which causes the recruitment of reserve muscle fibers in the target muscle. When the target is stretched with a reverse movement, the nervous system receives an emergency-response signal, and the muscle is put in an emergency state—reserve muscle fibers are called to action, which means more of the target muscle is stimulated to grow. Stretch overload also increases anabolic hormone release in lean muscle tissue. Examples: Incline pushups (chest), stiff-legged press (hamstrings) and neck presses (upper-traps).

CONTRACTED: Contracted: Here you place the target muscle in the most advantageous position for it to contract. These exercises have continuous tension, so they are perfect for blood-flow blockage, for a unique muscle-building response. Examples: leg curls (hamstrings), extensions (thighs), Liederman (chest).

A few other things to remember. First, during a set to exhaustion, low-threshold muscle fibers, fire first followed by higher-get-big-fast-twitch fibers. Those higher-threshold fibers are the most conducive to muscle-building-enhancement, and you only get to them by extending the tension time—more stress to the muscles, the more 2Bs you recruit; so volume is essential because each set brings in only a small number of those key growth fibers at the end. That's why the more you put into anything the more you grow.

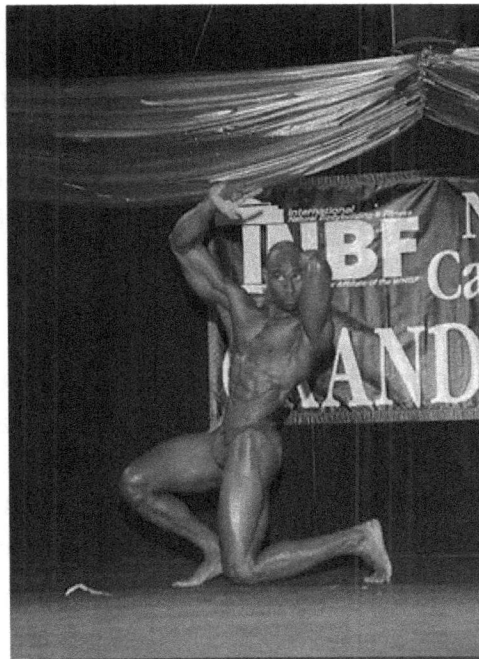

CHAPTER 2
INCREASING THE ANABOLIC COMPONENT

After my initial phase one and two experiments, I developed a number of stress methods and techniques, and with those my results soared again, as I added a few pounds of muscle. One of the best stress method for increasing the stress on the muscle fibers, is the, **TEN BY TEN METHOD** and **DOUBLE IMPACT**. That's performing a full rep followed by a half rep at the important stretch point between each full range rep. For example, on a bicep curl you pull the arm all the way up lower the arm to the bottom position, then pull it up to just below the half way point, lower to the beginning again, then pull the arm up towards the shoulders again. So you use a half rep between each rep in the set. Why is this method so special? It provides, greater force production on the muscles for optimal fiber-stimulation, the stretched point at the bottom of the movement. That (special) turnaround position is the "key" position for increasing growth stimulation.

The Double Impact action is a unique semistretch-point stimulus—but what happens when you adapt? A slight volume increase will ignite a new burst of sculpted muscle growth and strength. Enter **ISOMETRIC/PAUSE TRAINING** Isometric/Pause Training, When you reach exhaustion on your Double-Impact set, pause at the heightened position of the exercise stroke for 20 seconds. When you adapt to that, you can try another hybrid stress method within another phase. Got the idea?

In order to promote an efficient training protocol the trainee must mix and match various intensities and techniques to promote on-going improvements.

PARTIAL-ONLY SETS: INCREASE FIBER ACTIVATION AND TENSION OVERLOAD

So if the turnaround position is the best spot on an exercise stroke for fiber activation, why do any full reps at all? That's a Good question. We need full range reps as well, however, to keep the tension time on the muscles and increase fiber overload to turn on the hypertrophic process. Getting at least 30 seconds of target-muscle overload within that particular spot is necessary to "coax" muscle growth. That's why partial reps done by itself or, end-of-set partials are so powerful—the muscles keeps firing and it coax optimal-muscle-coaxing-stimulation.

ISOMETRIC PAUSE OVERLOAD TRAINING:

With Isometric Pause-Overload-Training you perform a certain amount of reps then pause for a count of 20 at the strongest muscle-stimulated position. (hence the term "overload"), and you do only Partial reps at the turnaround semistretch position. At one point I realized how important that type of maximum muscle stress is for growth, similar to that produced by forced partial reps, by itself to increase overload. So, isometric pause coupled with stretch overload created gains in muscle size that "surpassed previous expectations of the time required to acquire increased gains." (I got bigger faster!)

CHAPTER 2

ISOMETRIC-PAUSE TRAINING MUSCLE DEVELOPMENT AND DETAIL: Theres a number of reasons I've found why partial reps in the turnaround position build larger muscles quickly—everything from extended tension times to fast-twitch fiber activation to anabolic hormone surges. Experimenting I've come across some intensity methods that further enhance the muscle-morphing power of half reps, either between or Partial-Only. "Partial-range reps in the lower range of a muscle, will add sarcomeres to a muscle fiber, which would fill out the area of a muscle where it is inserted." I believe that may be a big reason I have made such dramatic improvements progress quickly that first time I integrated partials at the end of some of all my exercises—adding sarcomeres to muscle fibers creates much more muscle size, strength and muscle detail.

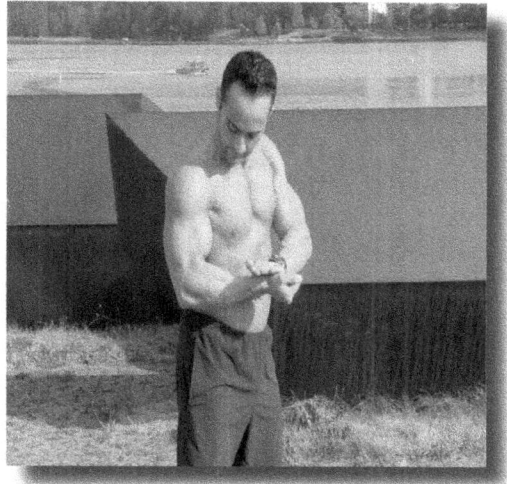

I have harped a lot on the importance of the semistretch position, the point at which the target muscle is somewhat elongated for optimal fiber activation. I have suggested that the partial position, is the ideal point for partials to engage more fibers. However, building fiber size through max-coaxing generation is only one layer of muscular development (albeit the primary one for most trainees). Other training protocols can add more layers for significant muscle-sculpting increases, such as blocking blood flow (occlusion). That means the appropriate partial spot depends on which size-building layer you're attacking with an exercise. Let me explain... The turnaround, where you move from the negative to the positive, is the generating-force point, so it makes sense to do partial reps there on most exercises like curls or decline-pushups.

CHAPTER 2

Those exercises moves—are specifically geared to force-generation fast twitch activation, so moving to the target muscle's semi-stretch point when you reach muscle fatigue full-range exhaustion amplifies force overload. (You fully know that because I've said it about 15 times now!) You use contracted position exercises, like concentration curls or tricep pushdowns, primarily to finish off the muscle with continuous tension, which blocks blood flow for occlusive hypertrophy. That's the goal for those exercises— continuous tension/occulsion—as they are best for building the muscle-coaxing-endurance components, like capillary beds and mitochondria, for more muscle size.

Now, the flexed, or contracted, position is where the target muscle is less capable of firing because the fibers are bunched up; remember, it's at elongation, the partial position, where they are properly aligned. That fiber bunching, like the top of a concentration curl, is not the best position for certain exercises. However, it is excellent for lateral raises additonal occlusion with partial reps because when you move to the bottom of the stroke, the semi-stretch point, it's easier to dis-engage the target muscle, and allow some blood to enter. So besides the midpoint of an exercise stroke, partials in the contracted (flexed) position appear at times to be best for triggering more occlusive hypertrophy.

At the beginning of my first experiment, I've tried the partial rep of each exercise at various ranges of motion per muscle designation. For example, partials for curls, the basic move, were performed from below to the middle of the exercise stroke; and for concentration curls were performed at the top, flexed position. Those earily points within my experiments eventually led me to many stress methods variations that improved my physique considerably. .
As I've mentioned, the year after my initial experiment I continued to research muscle growth and developed a number of methods and strength-coaxing techniques.

One of the best for contracted-position exercises, like concentration curls, was the **TEN, TEN, TEN METHOD**. It takes some pain tolerance, but you get the best of both worlds—occlusive growth stimulation followed by a bit more muscle-coaxing-force fast-twitch activation at the very end of the set. If you haven't read beyond Self Resistance books, here's how to use the method: Perform 10 full reps, followed by 10 reps from the bottom range to the half way mark, followed by another 10 full reps. The partial reps further occlude the biceps, while the full reps allow you to blast out the last bit of force from the fast-twitch fibers left standing—and you get a much longer tension time over-load. That's a serious dose of muscle stimulating—efficiency-of-effort muscle sculpting!

CHAPTER 2

DOUBLE IMPACT STRESS METHOD:
The Double Impact Overload technique, is a half rep in the semi-stretch position—the negative-positive turnaround—between each full rep. As mentioned earlier, that's the best place for max occlusion, so that's why I say emphasize it on these positions. This gives you even more growth-promoting tension time and you're able to squeeze out a bit more fiber activation. However you must have a high pain tolerance. It's all about stressing the muscle as much as you can to coax the muscle building progress......

ARE FULL REPS EVEN NECESSARY?
If (partial) half reps are best for blood blockage, and the half mark position is the optimal spot for maximum blockage, why do full-range reps at all? Also, what about the top part of the exercise contracted position? Why not just hold and flex the target muscle for an extended period of time to max out the occlusive growth effects even greatter muscle building stimulation?

I've experimented with that years ago and got great gains using static holds, although I didn't know about occlusive hypertrophy at the time (I simply figured I am hitting more fibers in the contracted position, but the key growth-inducing component of these exercises is bloodflow blockage). I adopted that style of training because I love Isometric training, and did a lot of **STATIC-CONTRACTION AND ISOMETRIC PULSES** experiments. Most times the holds were 20-60 seconds and I received a significant muscle increase and developed fantastic muscle detail by holding the contracted and mid-point positions of certain exercises, like the mid-point of a Liederman Press, for 40 seconds, at times increasing the tension or keeping the force at 30 percent and holding it for 60 seconds at times.

Most recently I have done another experiment on static-hold, Isometric contraction training. Using between six to nine exercises for three sets each, as a static hold for 20 to 30 seconds, the gains in enhanced muscle shape and defination was increased threefold—after only 15 days. And that's only static contraction training only! So does that mean you should only do static holds at the half mark contracted positions only? No, not if you want to optimize every facet of muscle growth, overload and tension/occlusion at various positions and exercises—so you look like a natural bodybuilder.

Attacking all of these components will transform your physique quickly by covering all of the muscle-building bases. However, those static-contraction trials do emphasize the flexed mid-point and contracted-position exercises in your workouts has significant muscle-building benefits—because it's the prime spot for triggering occlusive hypertrophy. So back to the question: Do you need full reps at all? I believe that you to a point, but you should do at least one or two full-range sets on your exercises. Why? Different muscle fibers fire throughout an exercise's stroke.

CHAPTER 2

If the trainee only train one spot within the stroke, you may not activate as many fibers as you could have. Plus, there's muscle-fiber recruitment patterns, firstly, you begin firing the slow-twitch fibers at the beginning of the set when the reps are easy, then toward the middle of the set you begin activating the fast-twitch type 2As, then at the end of the set, when the reps are hard, you finally bring in the type 2Bs, which are most conducive to growth. But wait! Didn't I say that the primary reason for partial mid-point reps is occlusive hypertrophy not fiber activation? Yes, but fiber activation is a secondary benefit of contracted-position exercises, so it shouldn't be ignored or you miss that muscle-growth component. In fact, all of the positions—muscle-teamwork, pre-stretch and contracted—can activate different fibers due to unique angles of pull or push.

That is why I suggest doing at least one or two sets of each through a full range. You want to irritate all "layers" of muscle growth. The bottom line for self resistance exercises: Do your first set with full-range movement. You can do the second set with a 20-30-second occlusive static hold at the mid-point position, or contracted position. That static-hold technique will help maximize occlusive hypertrophy, the primary growth stimulus of these important exercises and stress methods.

PRE-STRETCH EXERCISES:
PRE-STRETCHING AND FASCIAL LOOSENING

If you've read my other books, you know that stretch overload is a very special and powerful coaxing-get-big-trigger. Fully elongating a muscle with self resistance along with stress methods has been linked to everything from muscle-fiber expansion to anabolic hormone release. Stretch-position exercise, like decline pushups for the chest and lateral presses for the traps, also have the power to stretch and open up the fascial sheetings, the protective layer that encases muscle tissue. In truth, the fascial sheeting can constrict muscle growth if it's not stretched—you need to somehow make it more pliable so the muscle fibers and growth-enhancing contituents will expand further. As I have said, pre-stretch- exercises do help make the fascia more pliable to a degree.

In my books I have suggested performing a pause at the pre-stretch exercise before the turna-round begins for 5-10 seconds at a time. This increases the pump within the upper chest; so why not hold to stretch the fascial sheeting to promoted added growth? It is an excellent muscle-boosting strategy—but there may be a quicker more efficient way. If you perform a pre-stretch and contracted exercises and superset them, you can get a big pump and extreme fascial expansion in a matter of seconds while still getting the other anabolic benefits from those movements—tension/occlusion and stretch coaxing effects.

CHAPTER 2

For example: Start with one or two sets of incline pushups (muscle-teamwork for muscle-coaxing). Now comes the **FASCIAL-EXPANSION-SUPERSET**—decline pushups immediately followed by Liederman presses, rest for ten seconds, then blast through a second superset. The occlusion you get from the Liederman presses heightens blood blockage and muscle engorgement immediately within the set. The pre-stretch action of both the decline pushups and Liederman presses will be even better at pushing out the fascia, making it more pliable.

A second and even a third round, will add even more blood in your chest muscles, this will heighten the fascia-stretching action. Fascial expansion is a powerful technique for coaxing and unleashing new muscle growth. This focuses on coaxing-force generation, with focused pre-stretching bodyweight (muscle-teamwork) and self resistance exercises which gives you a greater pump with higher reps along with fascia expansion.

Obviously, fascial expansion is somewhat theoretical, but if nothing else, reversing the order and doing supersets will produce a fiber-recruitment-pattern change that will result in greater muscle-enhancing-gains. However, it is still almost as effective as the fascial-expansion superset because you still reverse the order of the two exercises—you get a big pump via occlusion with the contracted-or pre-stretch-position exercise (decline pushups/across the body press—you can do the second set in static-hold fashion, as explained—30-second hold in the contracted position, increasing the tension time to 60 seconds), then, after a few seconds of rest, you go to a stretch position exercise (liederman press) while the pecs are still full and throbbing. Just try not to rest too long after your decline sets to hit your first set of Liedermans or across the hip contracted movement. You don't want the pump to dissipate.
In the program I have included fascial expansion supersets; however, there is still that one nagging question...

ARE FULL REPS NECESSARY ON PRE-STRETCH EXERCISES?
If stretch-position exercises, like Declines for the chest and three-chair-dips for the lats, stimulate muscle growth via stretch overload, why not just hold the stretch position, like static holds on basic-stretch and contracted-position exercises? What I did was, hold the position in the stretch position on exercises like Liedermans and three-chair-dips to get that important growth stimulus? Perhaps, now on static contractions, for contracted-position movements there is a secondary mass-building characteristic involved that occurs with full-range reps.

CHAPTER 2

With stretch-position exercises it is additional targeted-force-output, the same key hypertrophic stimulus you get on muscle-team-work exercises (like thigh rowss and one legged squats). Now, "If a muscle shortens immediately after a stretch, two things happen 1)force and power output increases, and, 2)energy expenditure decreases. Thus, muscles can produce greater mechanical force and power while using less metabolic energy." That force/power translates into more endurance-fast-twitch muscle fiber activation.

So to get those muslce-coaxing-force-generation growth effects with stretch-position exercises, do your first set with near full range movement. On your second set you can use the **STRETCH-PAUSE** technique: Between reps pause for a count of 10-second hold in the stretch position; increase the static stretch for 20-30 seconds to increase and coax muscle-splitting to promote additional muscle growth.

PARTIAL REP TRAINING AND DOUBLE IMPACT:

I have done partial only sets with out-standing results. —Short, partial-range reps, usually starting near the semistretch point on the exercise stroke, was the dominant Birch size-tactic—and I've also used a lot of Double-Impact-Reps, in phases. Along with, high reps with long tension times dominate my workouts as well. Want specifics? I figured you will.

THE DOUBLE IMPACT/TEN BY TEN AND PARTIAL CHEST WORKOUT

I ran my very first workout on chest, and it took place 16 weeks out from the 2004 Mr. Universe contest. Don't think that because it's a full four months before the big show that I am out of shape. I was full, and still fairly vascular with separation, at a bodyweight of 185 pounds (along with abs). I started my chest workout with decline pushups feet on a stool hands on two blocks—and every rep of every set from the bottom position, the pre-stretched point, to about halfway up. It's rapid-fire partials all in a row.

I did a few reps, getting no fewer than 15—and at the end of most sets I did a number of shorter quarter reps; that is, single or double hitches near the turnaround point of the exercise stroke, before blasting up to the halfway point. This was my favorite stress methods and I used the same technique on three chair pushups, enhancing the pre-stretch on every set. Next up was Liderman presses, at times as opposed to full reps I did—every set through a partial range. My range on the Liedermans was more like two-thirds of the way across—pre-stretched to mid-point—so tension stays on the chest.

My rep count never go below 10, and my tension time: was 41 seconds; try it— Then on to various across the body and hip presses for the chest contracted position exercises. At times chair (dips) Charles Atlas style of 1920s my technique is interesting to keep the tension on the muscle I would pulse in the middle of the exercise stroke, never locking out or going to the point of pre-stretch. They're like middle range semi-partials. My sets were 3-4, getting anywhere from 15-20 reps—more extended continuous tension time on the already pumped-up chest muscles. The key fiber-activating pre-stretch point I am always yapping about.

CHAPTER 2

MASSIVE TRICEPS WORKOUT

Normally triceps are trained on a separate session from chest, my triceps is an interesting body-part to highlight—I have been told I've got some wicked full sweeping triceps. Firstly, I gradually turned up the heat, and warmed up the elbows, with a number of sets of tricep pressdowns—all top-range partials, never locking out. My reps are all over the map because the exercise is for warmup only: 20, 15, 25, 10. Very little rest between sets—normally 3-10 seconds then continue. My first exercise is decline extensions with elbows inwards.

All of my repetitions are from the bottom to mid-point, and on many of my sets I will use the hitching short-stroke double impact reps technique on the last few reps of a set. Apart from that it is forward tricep extensions starting off at the halfway mark on every rep—once again, all Half-Rep partials. My reps ranged from 20,15,12, ending with some semi-partial rep style hitches before the last few reps on some of those sets. After that it is three chair dips for partial-range reps, a few reps are performed in a pulsing motion through the middle portion range of the exercise stroke only, and this is done on all three sets for about ten pulses near the bottom—which was very far up from full stretch—prior to my last few reps.

The take-home message for trainees reading this manual is that partials are good on a number of different levels—continuous tension and fiber activation to be exact. Even partial only sets have their muscle-building place—as long as the rep counts are fairly high on the majority so tension time is long enough for extreme muscle-building-stimulation. As I have stated in my books, I have done this style of training for some time; and it's working quite well for me and a lot of self resistance trainees out there following these methods.

I've had many phone calls on trainees asking- what if they do partials exclusively on all exercises? Not a wise idea,—you need to maximize all the layers of growth, including anabolic hormone release. When a trainee develops enough force-production in generating fibers to fire rapidly they will have genetic superiority and other, anabolic benefits, which will make their workouts more precise. This manual can provide innovative techniques, not to mention motivation, that can help you increase lean muscle size—just don't go overboard, like trying to go full bore set for set, method after method. Go slow and easy and find your own groove after you've completed the full course or do the entire course again.
I highly recommend it.

CHAPTER 2

MORE ON MY TRAINING METHODS

•Onto the shoulder workout this begins with rear-delt upright rows. This is a hybrid move that stimulates the rear part of the shoulders, along with traps, mid-back and the side of the shoulders. You can see the medial and trap muscles working!

•For back I included a resisted pulldown/shoulder press, When performing this, to me it is best to lean backwards,that gives my upper-back muscles a bit of stretch and a better contraction, as the upper arms move into his sides. After across the body pulls, sometimes I did the first portion of the pull to mid-point.

•Prior to one legged squats I'd perform three to four high-rep sets of leg extensions with medium resistance. Reps were between 20-30. These lube up his knees and get lots of blood into his thigh muscles due to the occlusion effect produced by continuous tension.

•I would finish my bicep/forearm with hammer curls, or reverse curls to hit the brachialis, then regular palm up curls to the front, two sets, 15 reps.

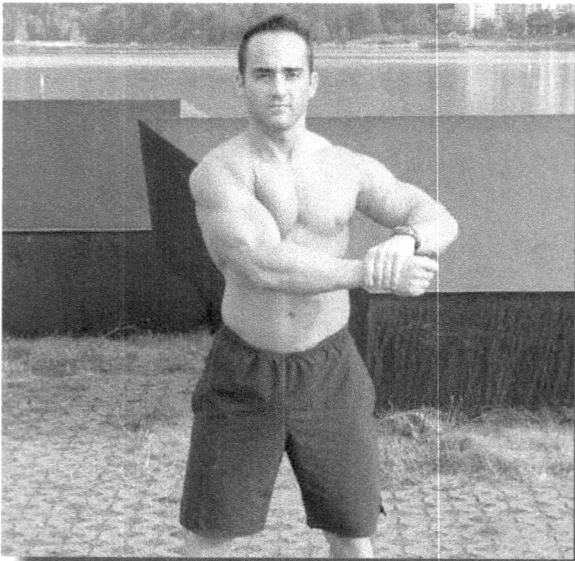

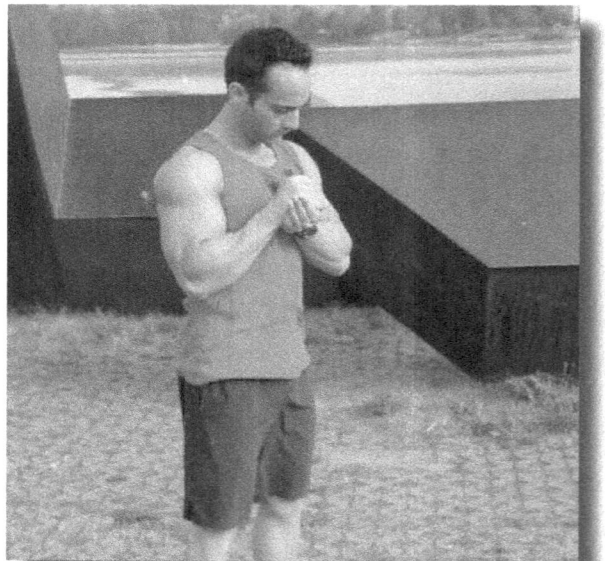

CHAPTER 3
MY AMAZING MUSCLE ENHANCEMENT EXPERIMENT

What happened is that I got much bigger than I'd ever been, so I gained at least 12 pounds of new muscle on the Muscle Enhancement program—and more on a second go of the system. As you will notice, the overall training scheme in the Serious Muscle Enhancement program is broken down into six-high-intensity training phases, the reason for the shorter-intensity 3 week phases is simple—the body adapts within a 4-6 week cycle. So to prevent full adaptation there is a back off so the body can handle more stress. When your body encounters a repeated form of stress like high-intensity strength resistance training, it will go through three levels of adaptation:

1) ADJUSTMENT PHASE: During the first week of training your body begin adjusting and gets weaker as it prepares to compensate for the new irritation being placed.

2) ADAPTATION PHASE: During the first three weeks your body actually adapts to the training irritation by getting larger and stronger.

3) HYPER-GROWTH PHASE: As the body continues to grow and get stronger due to new stimuli, no plateau takes place, and no regression will occur. By shifting into a different training module after three weeks of high-intensity training, you avoid adaptation entirely. In other words, you go from adjustment to adaptation, back to adjustment and then to adaptation again—you get continuous muscle-building coaxing effects, in a 18-week period.

Okay, let's look at the Muscle Enhancement Program...

Once again, the 18-week Muscle Enhancement training program is divided into six-high-intensity phases. Phase 1, listed on the next few pages, is a six-days-per-week routine that's designed to stimulate your natural testosterone production. But all of the workouts are not the same, as you will see. It is an innovative-but-tough program that make you work most bodyparts a few times per week—on Monday through Saturday, with the new and Improved stress methods and workouts.

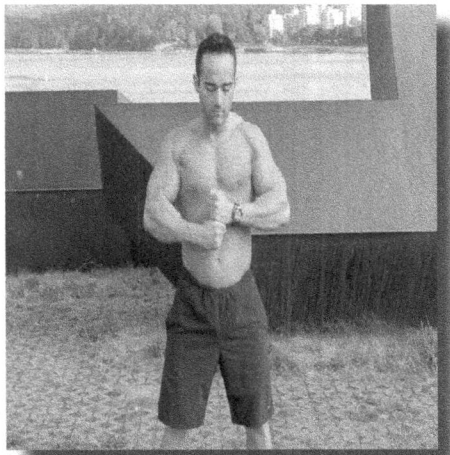

SERIOUS MUSCLE ENHANCEMENT WORKOUT 23

CHAPTER 3

THE ORIGINAL PHASE ONE WORKOUT
PERFORM THIS ROUTINE FOR 4 WEEKS FULL REPS ONLY

Day One
Decline Pushups
Liederman Presses
Crossed feet squats
Resisted leg extensions
Leg curls
Resisted pulldowns
Three chair dips
Across the body rows
Decline pushups (elbows out)
Resisted shoulder press
Resisted upright pulls

Day Two
Thigh rows
Standing calve raises
Reverse crunches
Across the body side crunches
Resisted forward tricep presses
Tricep pressdown
Bicep curl palm up
Reverse curls
Palm up wrist curls
Palm down wrist curls

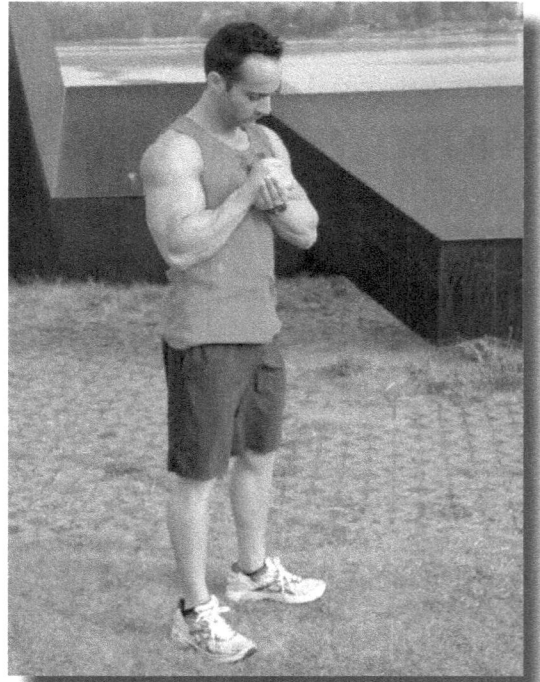

CHAPTER 3

Day Three
Crossed feet squats
Resisted leg extensions
Resisted leg curls
Standing calve raises
Decline pushups
Liederman presses
Resisted pulldown
Across the body rows
Decline pushups (elbows out)
Resisted shoulder press
Resisted upright pulls

Day four repeat day two and continue the routine as follows till day six. Rest on day seven.

Week One: 3 sets each exercise, 15 reps bodyweight 15 reps resistance moves.
Week Two: 4 sets each exercise, 20 reps bodyweight 10-12 reps resistance moves.
Week Three: 3 sets each exercise, 30 reps bodyweight 7-9 reps resistance moves.
Week Four: 4 sets each exercise, 15-25 reps bodyweight 15 reps resistance moves. At the mid point at the end of your self resistance moves, perform a isometric (static) hold for 20-30 seconds using moderate tension.

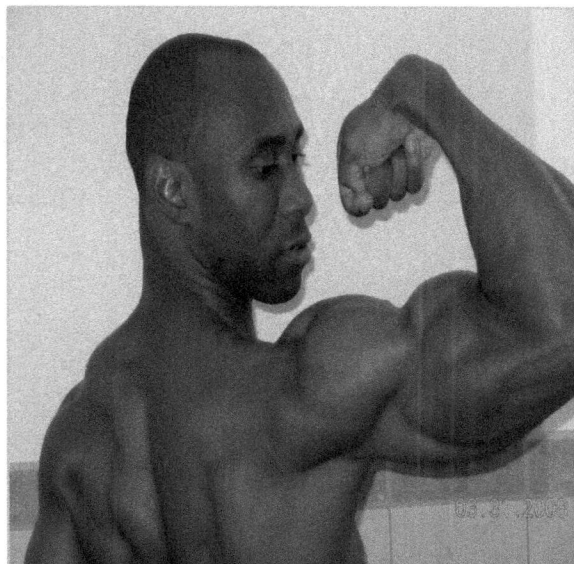

Results after the Hybrid round of the program with new stress methods

CHAPTER 3

THE ORIGINAL PHASE ONE WORKOUT
THE BEGINNING PHASE TWO

PHASE TWO 4 weeks
Day One

LEGS
One legged squats
Resisted leg extensions
Stiff-legged press
Resisted leg curls

CALVES
Slanted calve raises
Standing calve raises

UPPER CHEST
Decline pushups
Upper chess press

LOWER CHEST
Liederman press

TRICEPS
Resisted forward lateral press
Over head tricep press
Palm up tricep pressdown

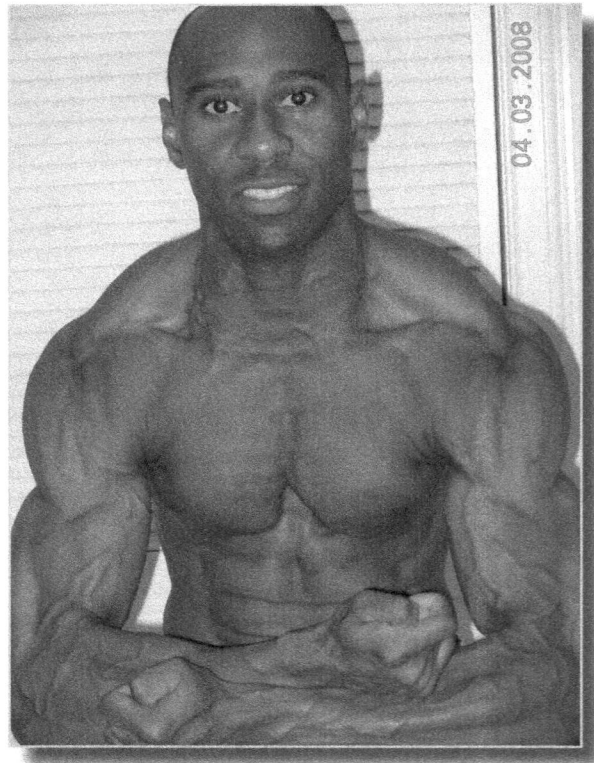

Marlon messing around

Day Two
UPPER BACK
Across the body rows
Three chair dips
Resisted pulldowns
Stiff arm pulldown

UPPER TRAPS
Rear neck press
Side to side neck press

SHOULDERS
Decline pushups (elbows out)
Across the body lateral raises
Resisted forward raises
Across the body pulls

BICEPS
Palm up curl
Hammer curl
Resisted concentration curls

ABS
Reverse crunches
Across the body situps
Across the body side crunches

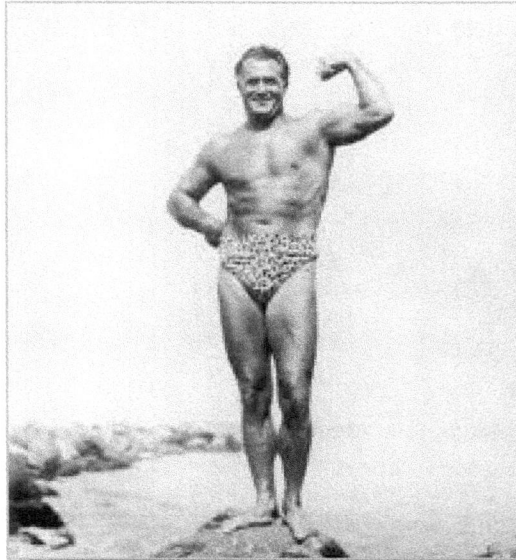

Marlon's Mentor Charles Atlas

Day one and day two are alternated throughout the week for 6 days of training. 3 sets each exercise. 20 reps bodyweight moves, 10-12 reps resistance moves. Continue this this phase for 4 weeks

CHAPTER 4

BODYPART ANALYSIS (EXPLANATION) NECK UPPER TRAPEZIUS EXERCISES

The neck muscles and upper trap muscles are the most important muscles in the body apart from the lower back. The neck is very important and supports the weight of your head that's 8-10 pounds. All the neck exercises increases the strength, size and shape to the neck. As we say in the fitness world, alinement starts at the top! A well rounded neck/upper traps routine will enhance one's posture and maintain balance for the head.

The neck muscles are incredibly important to train although most people ignore them. They shouldn't. A strong neck reduces the risk of injury and pain in this area. It can help reduce migraines and headaches as well as improve your posture. It can also improve the flow of blood to the brain, which will help keep you young. The neck development program that follows can help you with all of this..

CHAPTER 4

BODYPART ANALYSIS (EXPLANATION) NECK UPPER TRAPEZIUS EXERCISES

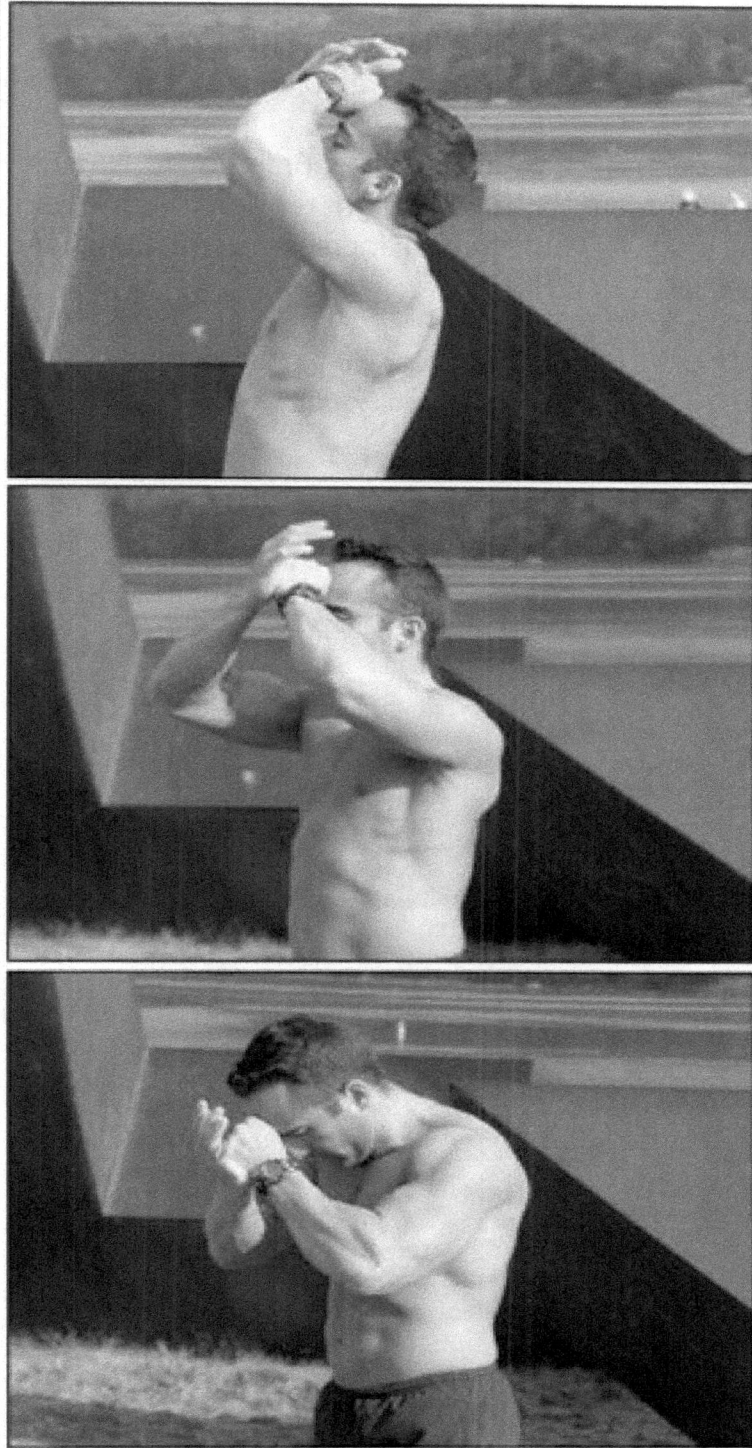

CHAPTER 4

BODYPART ANALYSIS (EXPLANATION)
NECK UPPER TRAPEZIUS EXERCISES

NECK AND UPPER TRAPEZIUS EXERCISES
Front Neck Press (Stretch and Contracted)

With your head tilted back place your hand on your forehead. Now slowly press your head forward and resist the movement slightly with light tension towards your upper chest. Always use a light tension to the neck. As your strength increases use a little more force but not too much tension. Breathe Normal.

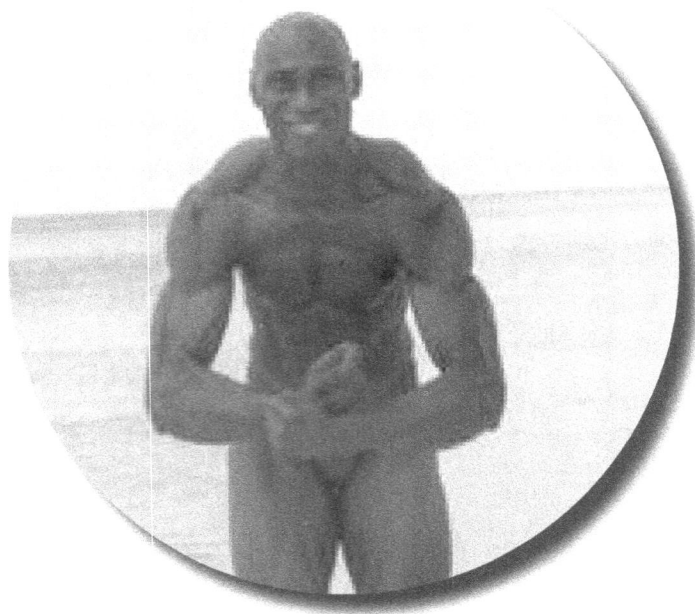

CHAPTER 4

BODYPART ANALYSIS (EXPLANATION)
NECK UPPER TRAPEZIUS EXERCISES

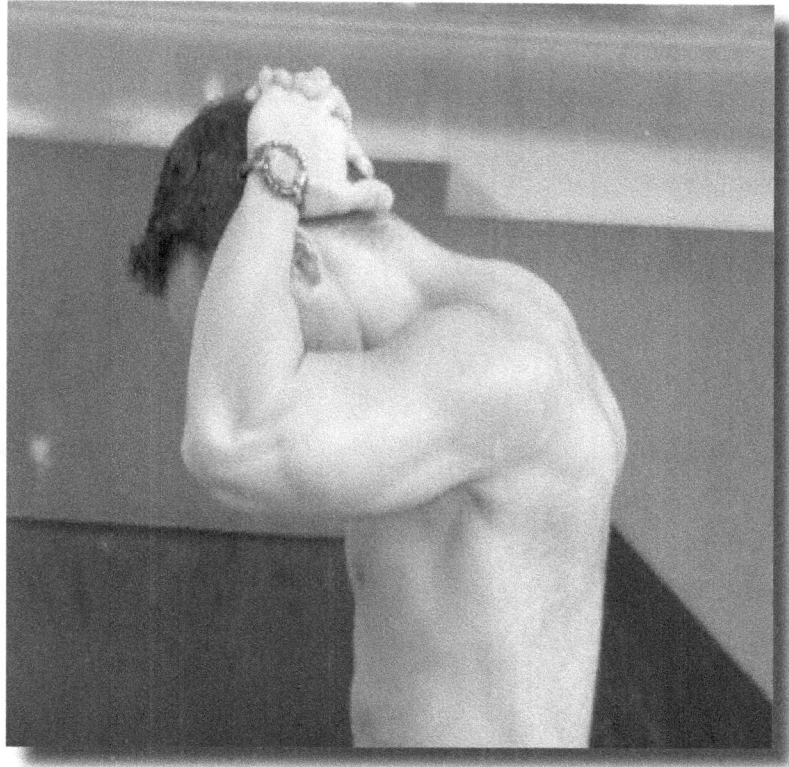

Rear Neck Press (Contracted)

CHAPTER 4

BODYPART ANALYSIS (EXPLANATION)
NECK UPPER TRAPEZIUS EXERCISES

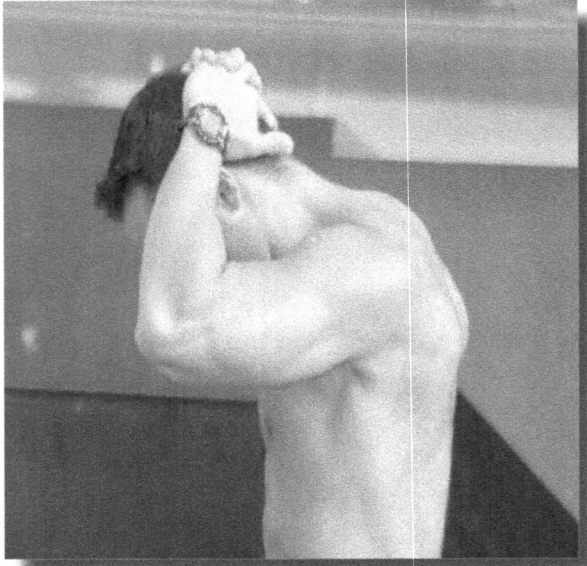

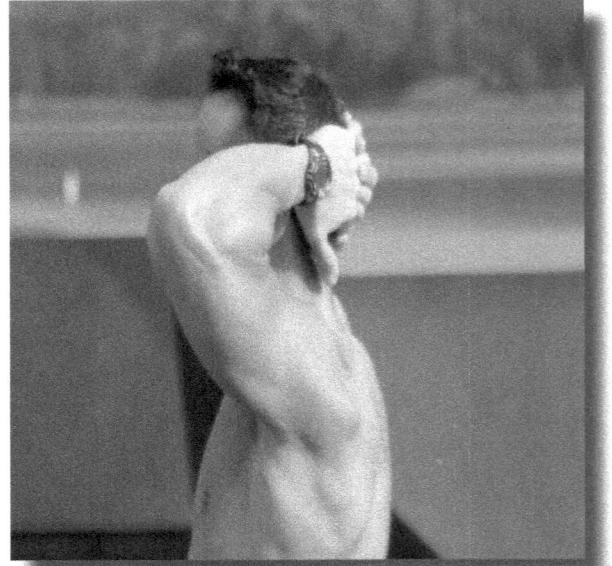

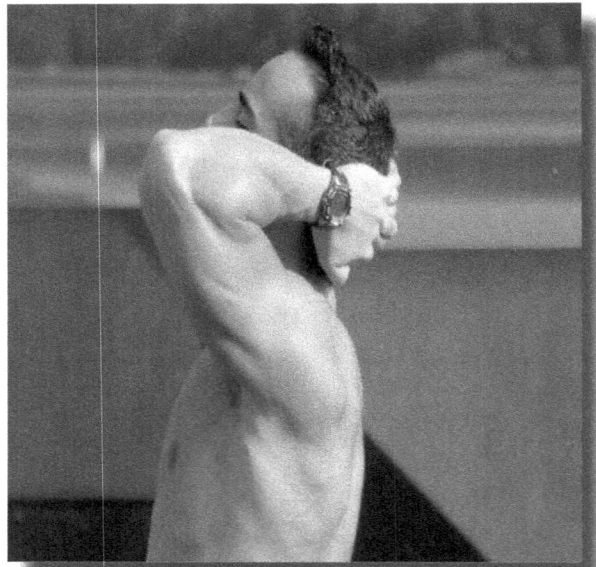

This movement is the opposite of the first movement. Place one hand behind your head and tuck the chin on the upper chest as shown. Now press the head against the hand while resisting with the hand until you're looking straight up. Use a light tension at the beginning and increase the tension to medium as you get stronger and more conditioned.

CHAPTER 4

BODYPART ANALYSIS (EXPLANATION)
NECK UPPER TRAPEZIUS EXERCISES

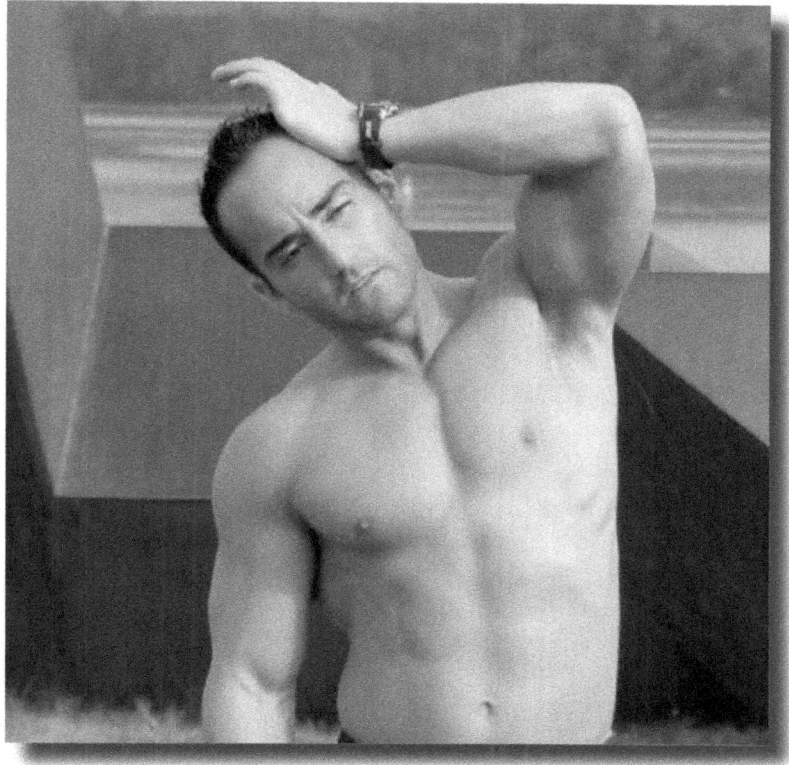

Side to Side Neck Upper-Trap Press (stretch)

CHAPTER 4

BODYPART ANALYSIS (EXPLANATION)
NECK UPPER TRAPEZIUS EXERCISES

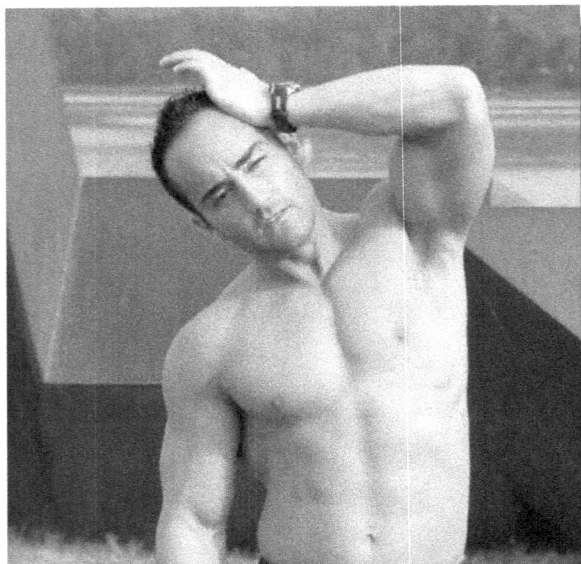

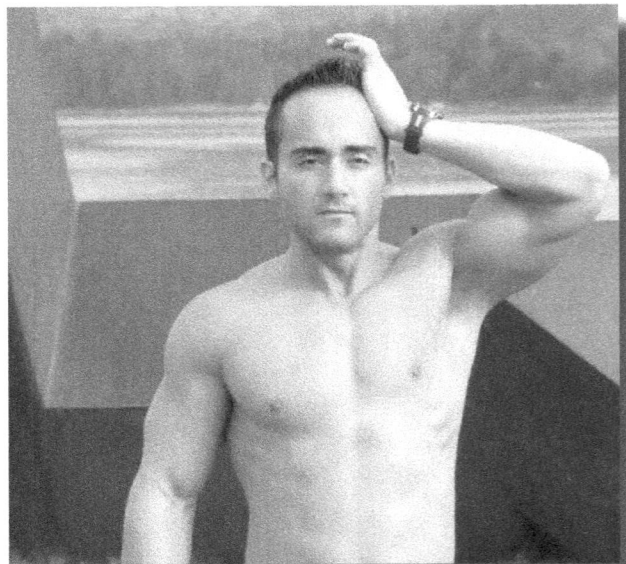

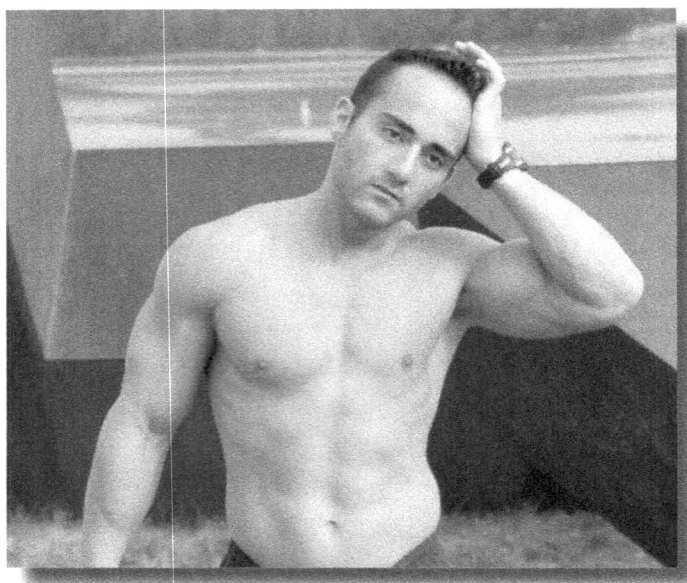

Bend your head as close as you can to the shoulder as shown. Place the left hand on the left side of the head and press the head to the opposite shoulder while resisting with the hand. Followed by placing the right hand on the right side and press the head back to the starting position as before. Dual action left then right. Remember use a light tension and once the neck becomes more conditioned and stronger increase the tension.

CHAPTER 4

BODYPART ANALYSIS (EXPLANATION)
CHEST EXERCISES

It's important to hit the chest muscles from many angles as possible to coax and force development. However, I learned that in order to really build a good chest it isn't one or two exercises it's a variety that will build the chest and increase it's strength! So in truth the best thing to do is to divide the chest in sections. Upper Chest, Inner Chest, Lower Chest. Instead of looking at it as a whole because it isn't. You must treat the upper and lower chest as two separate entities for your chest building venture to be a success.

In my early years I did loads of pushups for the chest which hits mostly the lower and outer portions of the chest and do next to nothing for the upper chest. So I switched to decline push-ups hands on blocks elbows in instead of out and the upper chest was taxed a great deal! So now my chest building starts with upper chest training. Giving priority to developing and stressing the upper chest.

Basic& Stretch: Decline pushups elbows in hands on a block works the upper chest really well. Along with help from the front portions of the shoulders and the tricep muscles.

Stretch& Contracted: Liederman Presses and Across the body presses really hit both elements in pre-stretching and increasing the peak contraction at the end of the movement. This position involves muscle-teamwork as well which will help the chest perform the movement. Help from the shoulders and triceps. Let's take a look at some muscle sculpting exercises.

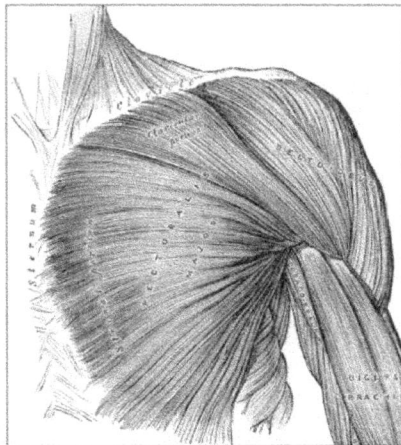

The purpose of the pectoral muscles is to move the arms downwards, forwards, and across the chest. These muscles greatly enhance one's physique and can greatly aide one's ability in all racquet and combat sports.

CHAPTER 4

BODYPART ANALYSIS (EXPLANATION)
CHEST EXERCISES

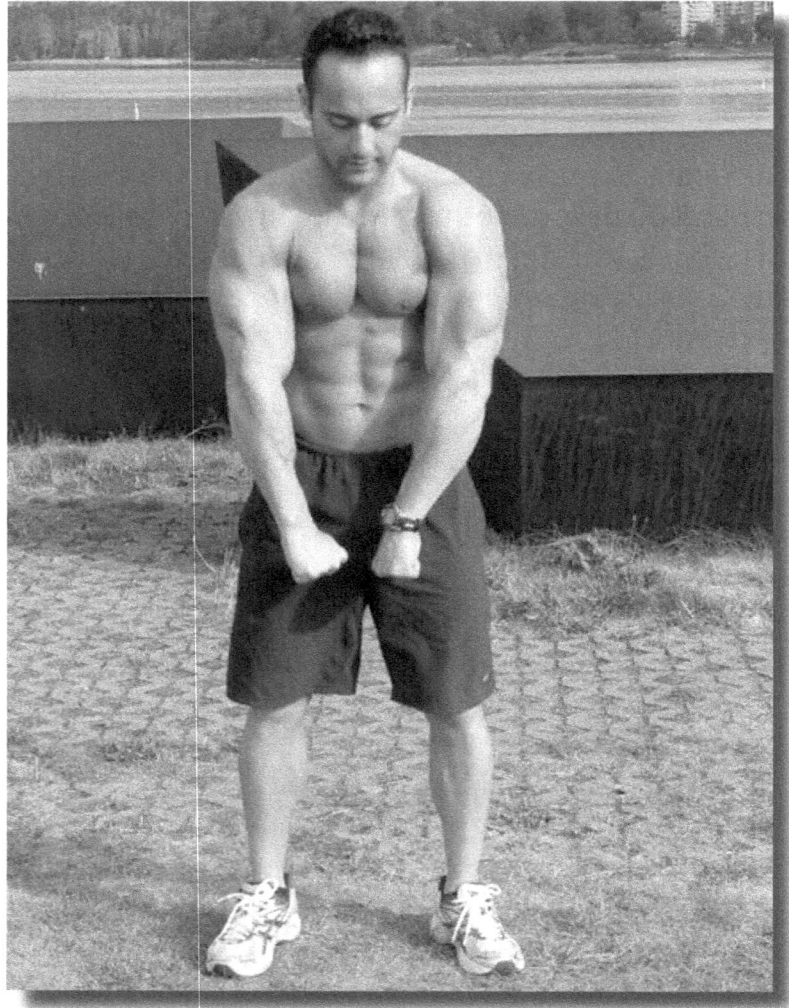

Chest Contraction

CHAPTER 4

BODYPART ANALYSIS (EXPLANATION)
CHEST EXERCISES

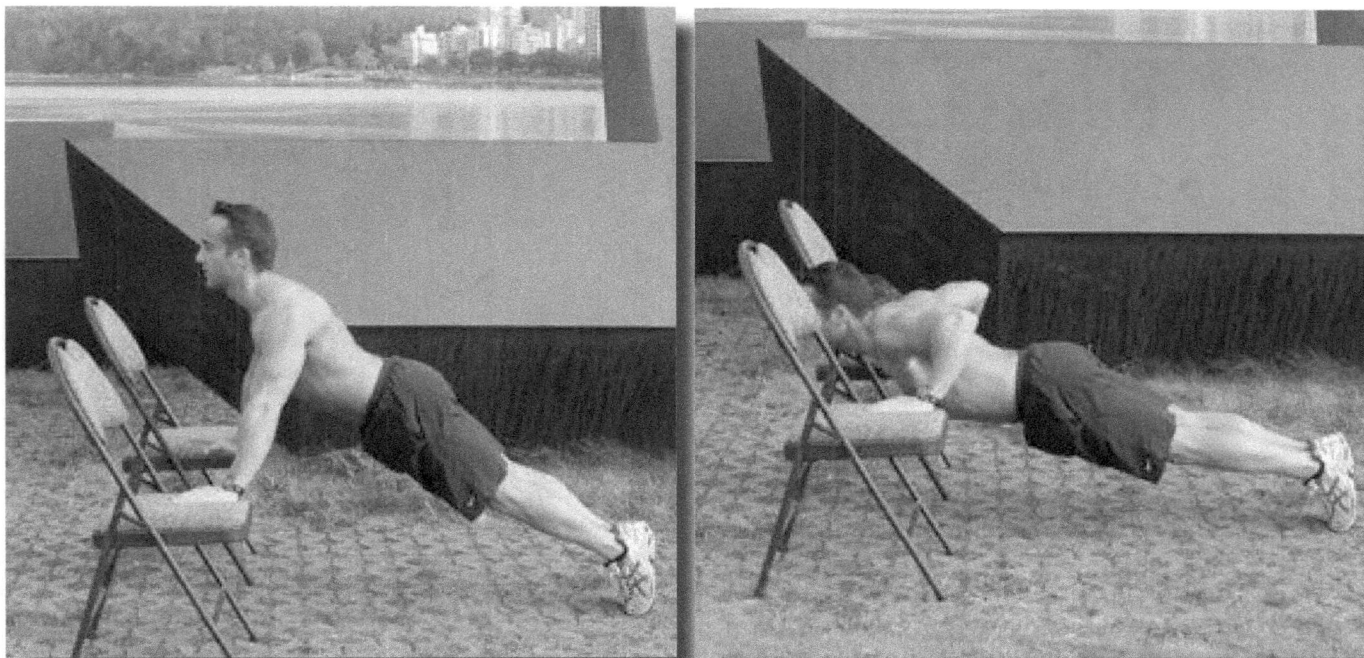

Incline Pushups (Basic and Stretch)

This exercise is the Granddaddy of all upper-body exercises. This was his key upperbody exercise for the chest. It's the best upper-body builder and conditioner there is. This exercise is performed exactly as shown. Place your hands two chairs or box that's10-15 inches high, the higher you go the greater pre-stretch there is. At the bottom position to enhance muscle building stimuli pause at the bottom for 2-3 seconds before reversing the movement. Excellent for the lower chest.

CHAPTER 4

BODYPART ANALYSIS (EXPLANATION)
CHEST EXERCISES

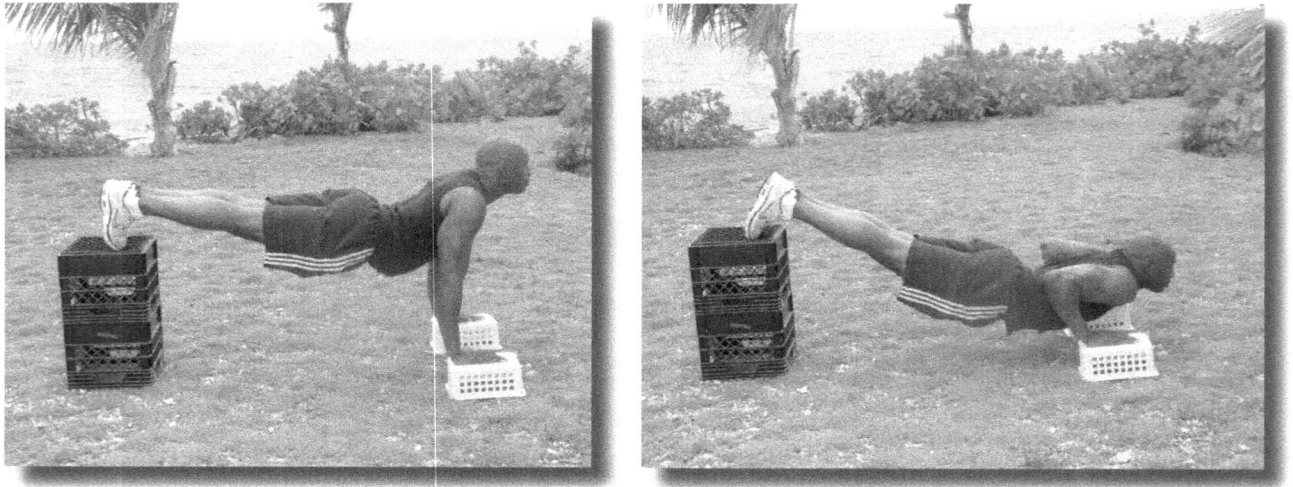

Decline Push-Ups (Basic and Stretch)

Another fantastic exercise is the decline pushups. An advanced version of the original Lieder-man pushup. This was his key upperbody exercise for the chest. It's the best upper-body builder and conditioner there is. This exercise is performed exactly as shown. Place your feet on a chair or box that's10-15 inches high the higher you go the greater pre-stretch there is. At the bottom position to enhance muscle building stimuli pause at the bottom for 2-3 seconds before reversing the movement. Excellent for the upper and lower chest.

CHAPTER 4

BODYPART ANALYSIS (EXPLANATION)
CHEST EXERCISES

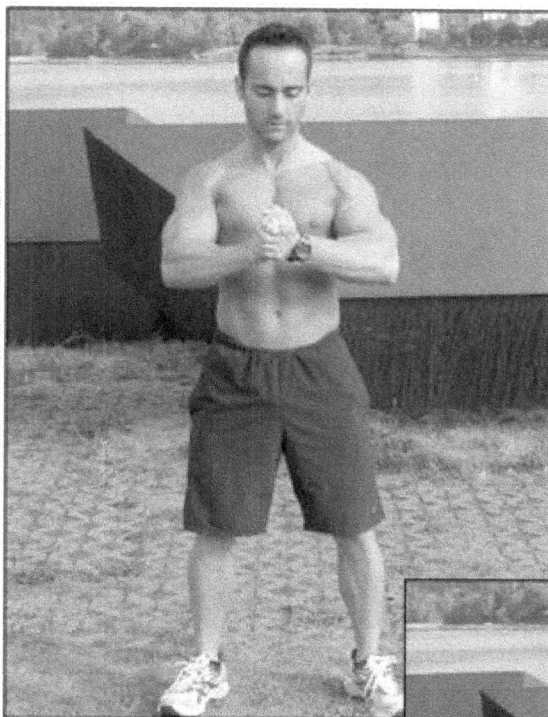

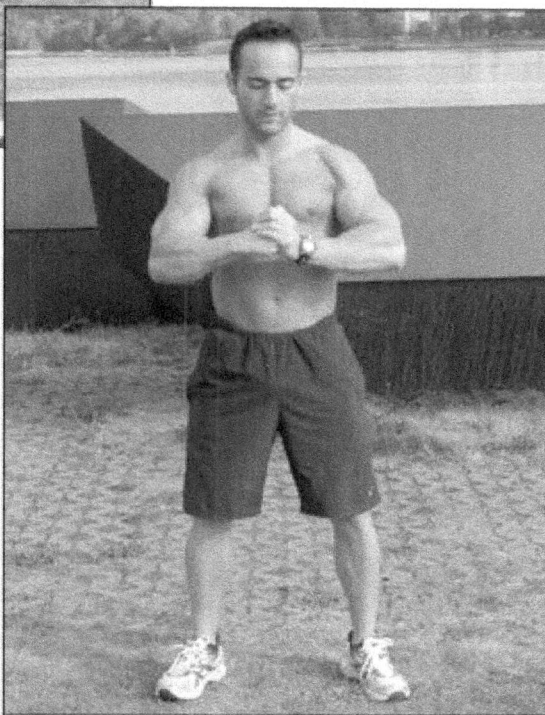

Liederman Press (Stretch and contracted)

This is an Awesome building and shaping movement. Works the entire chest, lower, upper and middle chest as well as the shoulders and tricep musculature.Start off with the hands as shown at the right armpit. Press right palm against the left palm towards the left armpit. Pause for 1-2 seconds

and press the arm back to the other armpit, pause again before repeating.

SERIOUS MUSCLE ENHANCEMENT WORKOUT 39

CHAPTER 4

BODYPART ANALYSIS (EXPLANATION)
UPPER BACK-MID TRAPS EXERCISES

The structures of the upper back is quite powerful every point needs to be very carefully targeted. Basic Synergy Muscle Team Work, works well here. Thigh Rows, Resisted Pull-downs or Three Chair Dips are major corner-stone exercises to target the powerful upper back muscles. This will be explained within this chapter

BACK ANALYSIS

The upper back is very complex and house loads of different muscles com larger areas of the back the lats, upper neck and mid back muscles. This will hit the smaller muscles as well.The best way to start is to break things down into sections to see where what is targeting to really realize what you're doing and how to effectively target that large mass of muscle more efficiently.

Strong, broad shoulders are considered desirable by both men and women. They can not only enhance your appearance but can also help you in any sport you play. The following exercises will help you build and sculpt your shoulders.

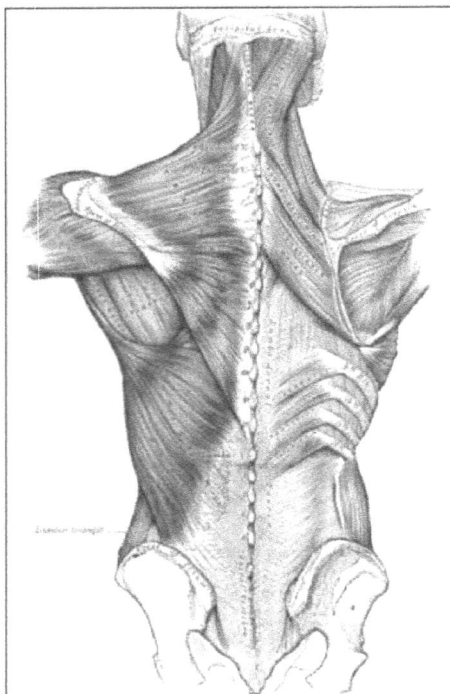

CHAPTER 4

BODYPART ANALYSIS (EXPLANATION)
UPPER BACK-MID TRAPS EXERCISES

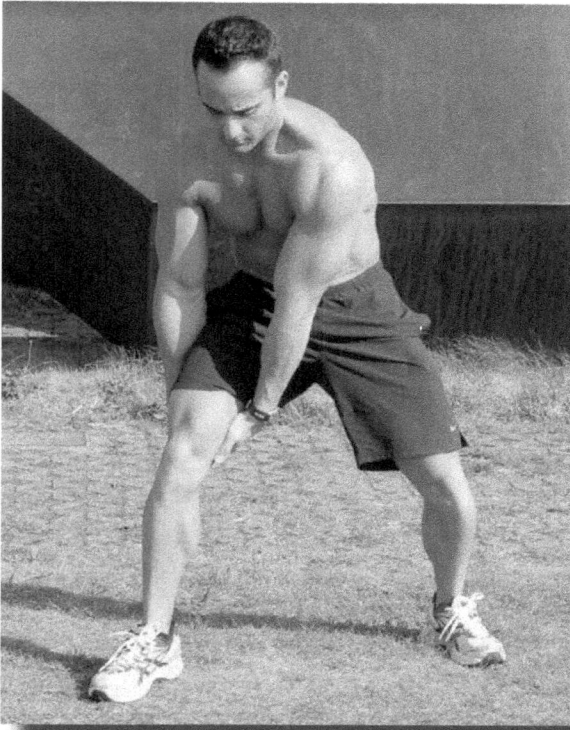

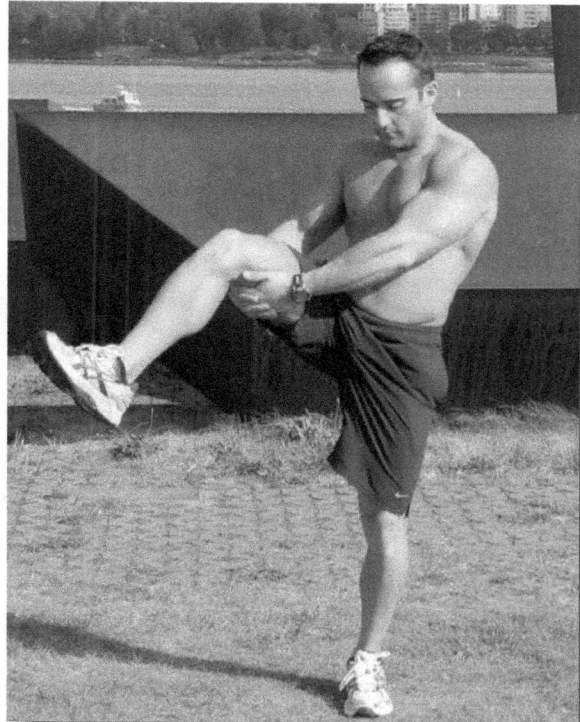

Thigh Rows (Basic)

Basic: Thigh Rows, these are perfect for targeting the upper and lower lat muscles as well as the lower back. Apart from that there's Resisted Pull-downs that targets the lats fully from top to bottom. These exercises are under continuous tension within the range of pull. However with the Thigh Rows resistance drops off a bit at the top position but by all means a highly effective exercise.

Interlock the fingers behind the knee as shown with right leg. With both arms pull the thigh up-wards towards the chest while resisting with the leg. This exercise widens the upper back, works the mid-back and stimulates the biceps as well. Work one side fully then switch to the other side. If balance is an issue perform the exercise seated.

CHAPTER 4

BODYPART ANALYSIS (EXPLANATION)
UPPER BACK-MID TRAPS EXERCISES

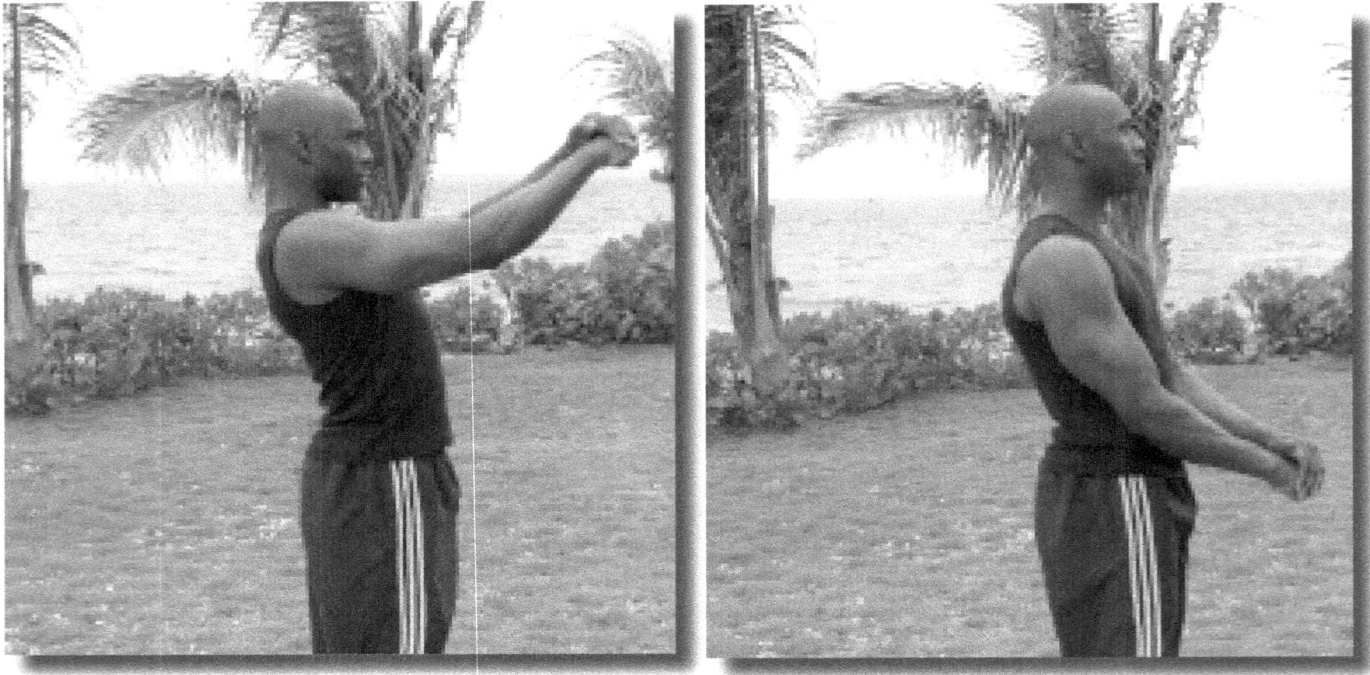

Stiff Arm Pulldown (Contracted)

Grasp the left hand with the right as in the picture. Gradually pull the arm downwards while resisting with the bottom arm. At finished position, Repeat by pressing the bottom arm up again by resisting against the top hand. Resisting in both directions for reps, then switch.

Fantastic Upper and mid back strengthener.

CHAPTER 4

BODYPART ANALYSIS (EXPLANATION)
UPPER BACK-MID TRAPS EXERCISES

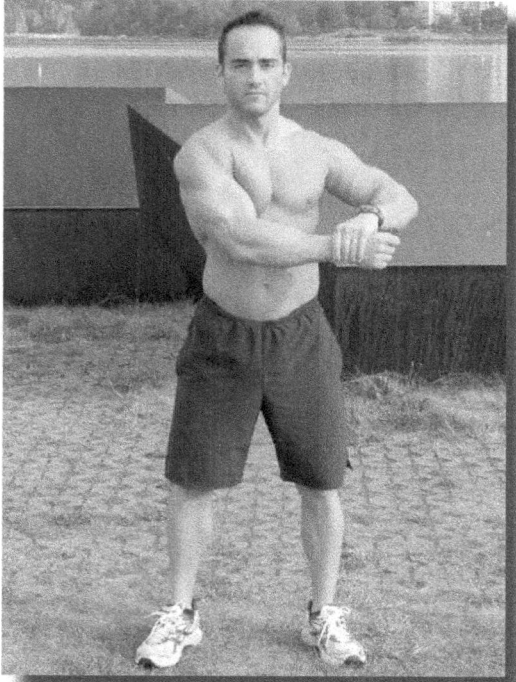

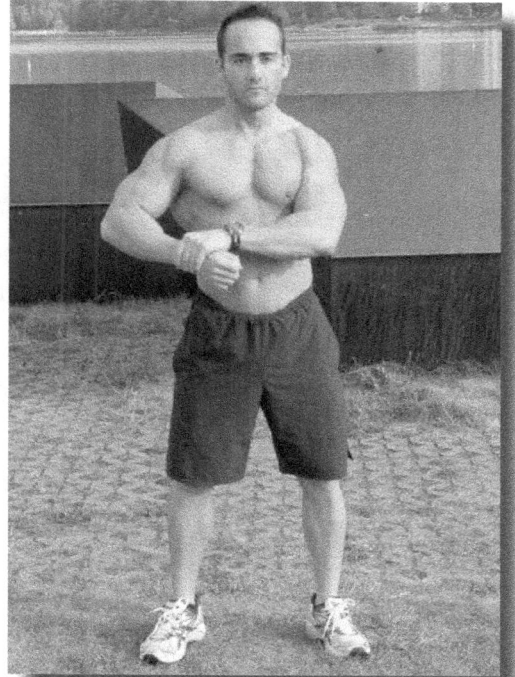

Across The Body Rows (Basic/Stretch/Contracted)

Bring your right arm across the body pre-stretching the mid-back, grasp the wrist with the left hand. Slowly pull the arm across the body toward the right armpit against the resistance supplied by the left hand. Repeat the movement then switch arms. This adds thickens to the mid back and lats, along with the rear part of the shoulders.

CHAPTER 4

BODYPART ANALYSIS (EXPLANATION) UPPER BACK-MID TRAPS EXERCISES

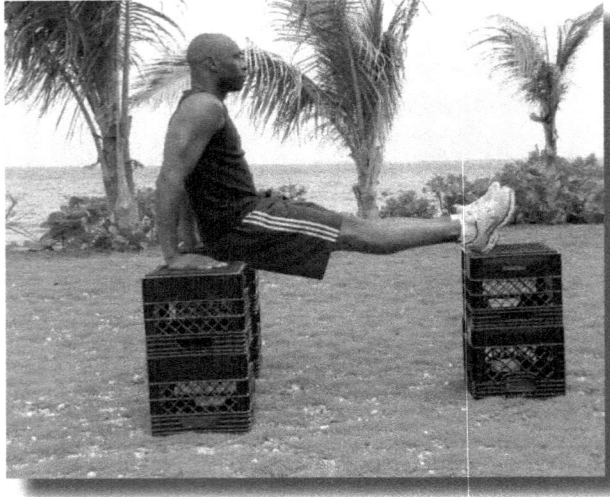

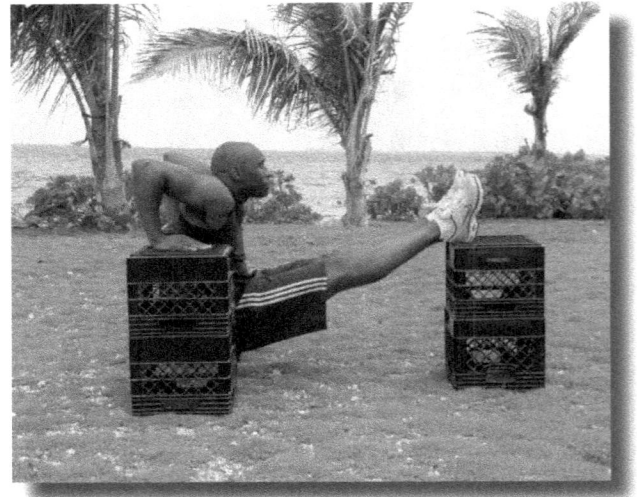

Three Chair Dips (Basic/Stretch/Contracted)

As shown place each hand at least 15-16 inches apart, or shoulder width. Lower the body between the chairs pause one second and reverse the movement to the starting position. This is an awesome upper back widener.

CHAPTER 4

BODYPART ANALYSIS (EXPLANATION)
UPPER BACK-MID TRAPS EXERCISES

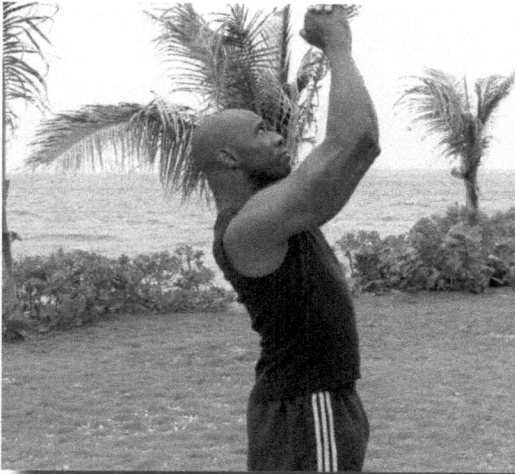

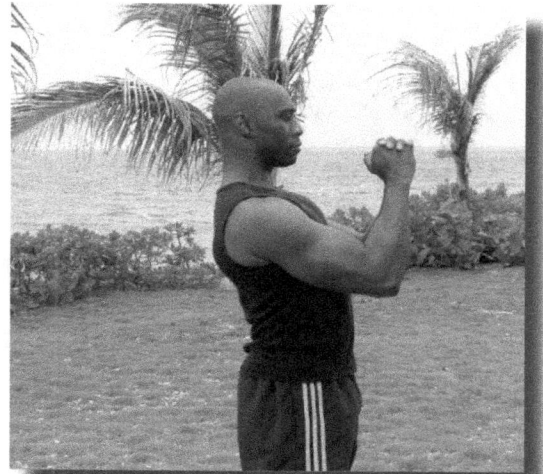

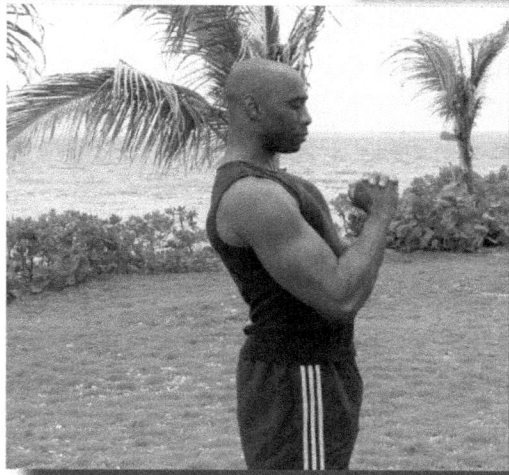

Resisted Pulldowns (Basic and Contracted)

With the arms overhead place your left hand on top of the right fist as shown. Pull down with the left hand resisting with the right, once at finished position press the right hand up resisting with the left hand for the desired reps. Then switch arms. This works the entire upper back, biceps, and shoulders

CHAPTER 4

BODYPART ANALYSIS (EXPLANATION)
UPPER BACK-MID TRAPS EXERCISES

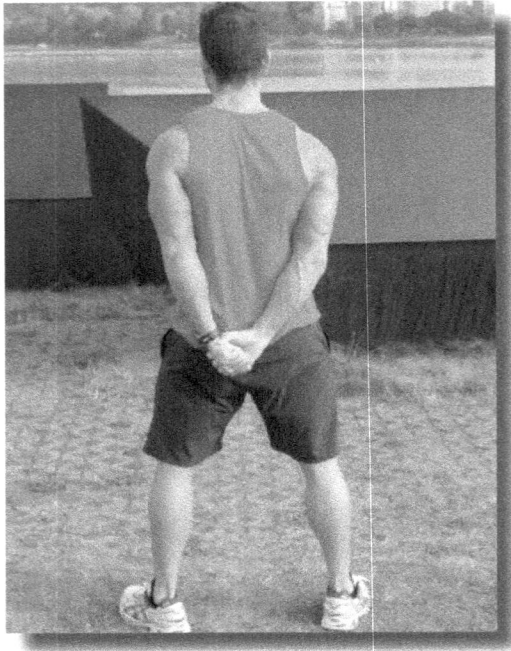

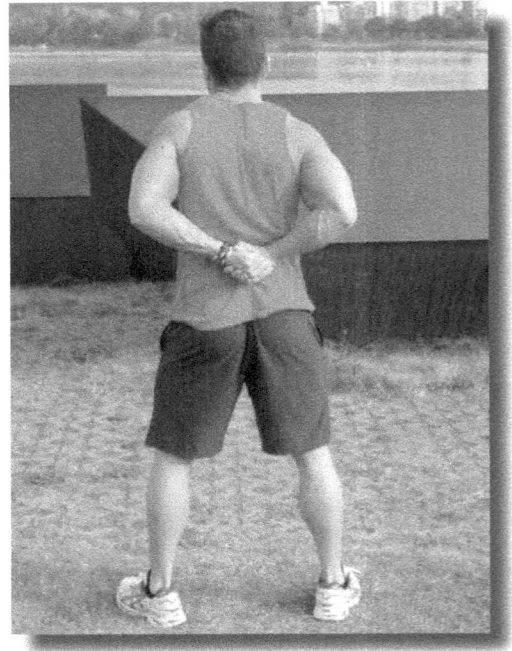

Reverse Upright rows (Contracted)

Place your arm behind your back as shown, hold onto the wrist with the other hand lean forward a-little and pull the right arm upwards while resisting with the right. When fatigue switch arms and continue. This works the mid-back,upper traps and rear delts.

CHAPTER 4

BODYPART ANALYSIS (EXPLANATION)
SHOULDER EXERCISES

There's exercises that directly target the side head of the shoulders giving you that wide look. However at the very start I did an exercise that was just magic in terms of side and overall muscle development and strength. It's decline pushups hands on floor (elbows out).

One can perform this by itself or with the isolation self resistance type exercises to add even more strength and muscle growth. Now it's been said that the lateral (side) will only be activated with lateral movements..but both forward and side resisted raises will stimulate the two heads.

The reason? One works with the other and they are intertwined with each other. The shoulder routine are packed with strength building and muscle pumping exercises that will create more width and roundness with efficient and muscle stimulating exercises. The shoulders contain three separate muscle heads, Front, Side and Rear heads. Lets take a closer look.

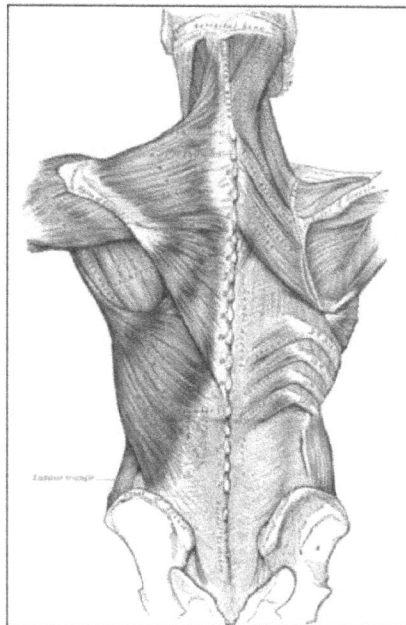

Strong, broad shoulders are considered desirable by both men and women. They can not only enhance your appearance but can also help you in any sport you play. The following exercises will help you build and sculpt your shoulders.

CHAPTER 4

BODYPART ANALYSIS (EXPLANATION)
SHOULDER EXERCISES

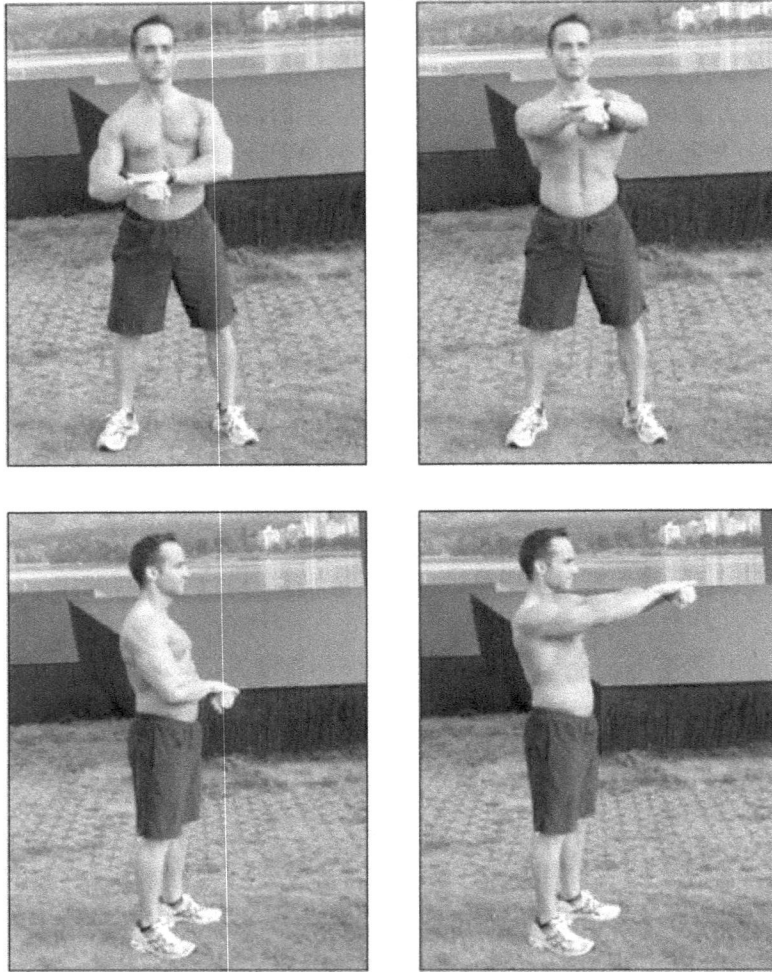

Forward raises

CHAPTER 4

BODYPART ANALYSIS (EXPLANATION)
SHOULDER EXERCISES

Now with all the pushing movements You'll be doing within this course you may think that you should lay off shoulder exercises a little seeing that almost all the upper body exercises contain some form of shoulder involvement.

The shoulders, just like the calves and forearms. Constantly working. Flexing and relaxing all day long when we walk, write/type, drive, lift a bag or put something on a shelf. Just like the upper back you need to separate the sum of parts and hit them in sections to really optimize your training when it comes to that area. Once separated precise and efficient training will surface.

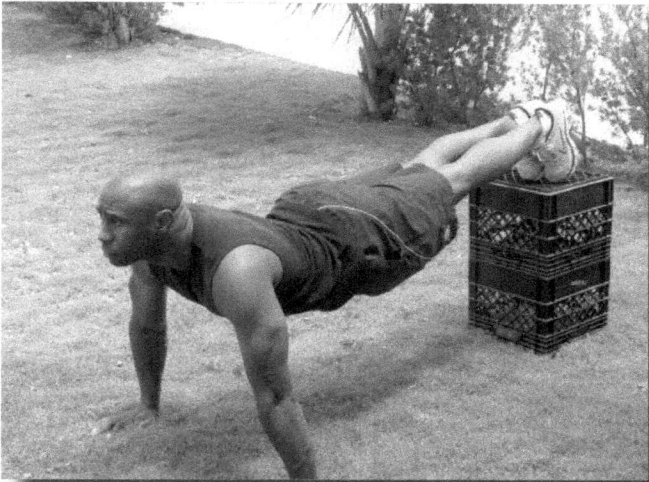

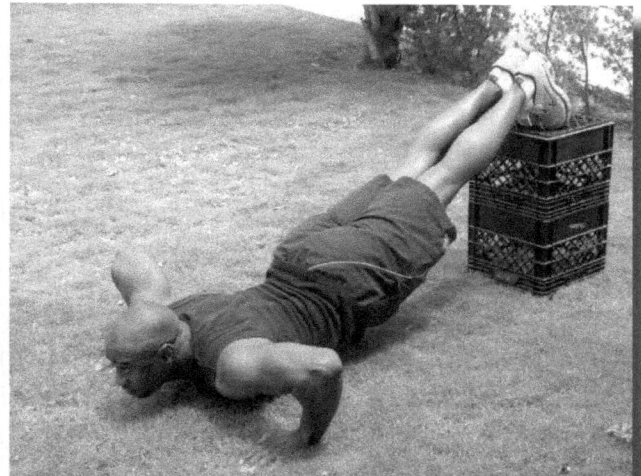

Decline Pushups (Basic)

The Liederman Pushups.... This exercise is performed exactly as above. Hands on the floor, feet on a chair or stool at least 15 inches or more, the higher the stool the more the shoulders and upper chest work. Lower yourself as close to the ground as possible, then press back up again.

CHAPTER 4

BODYPART ANALYSIS (EXPLANATION)
SHOULDER EXERCISES

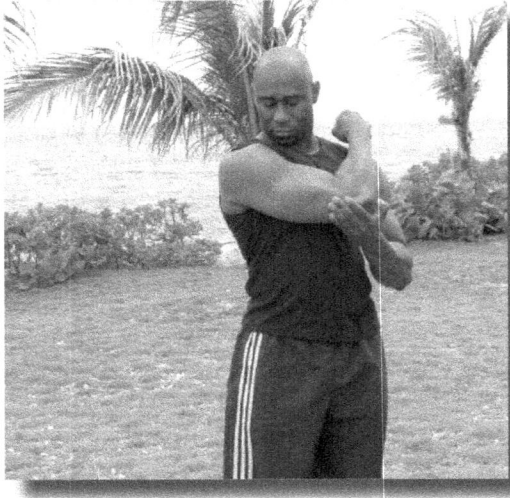

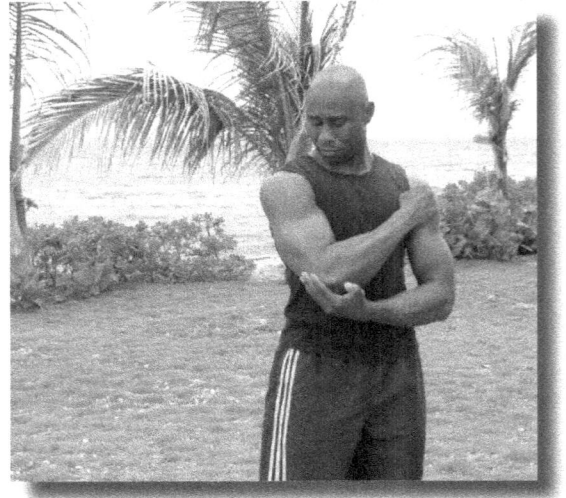

Across The Body Pulls Rear Delts (Contracted)

Grasp the right elbow as picture shows firmly with the left hand. Slowly force the right elbow downward and backward while resisting with the left hand. Repeat for reps, then switch arms. This add great strength and development to the (rear) back part of the shoulders, lats and mid-back. It's best to start with this exercise first for it's easily neglected in a muscle-building program. As they say, Out of site out of mind.

CHAPTER 4

BODYPART ANALYSIS (EXPLANATION)
SHOULDER EXERCISES

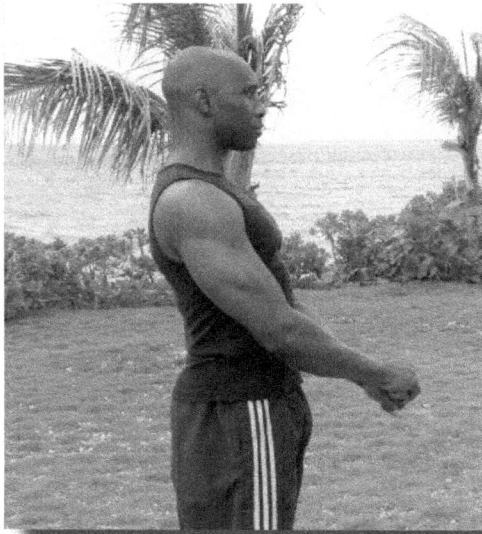

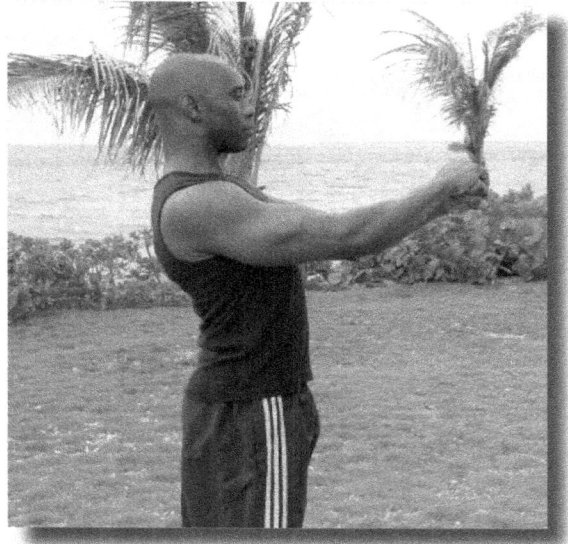

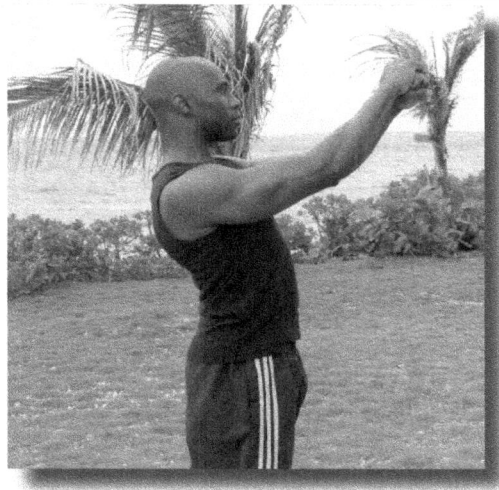

Resisted Forward Raises (Contracted)

Grasp the right hand with the left in front of the body as shown. Gradually raise the arm forward against the resistance of the other hand. Repeat for reps. Then switch arms and continue. This works the Front shoulder muscles.

CHAPTER 4

BODYPART ANALYSIS (EXPLANATION)
SHOULDER EXERCISES

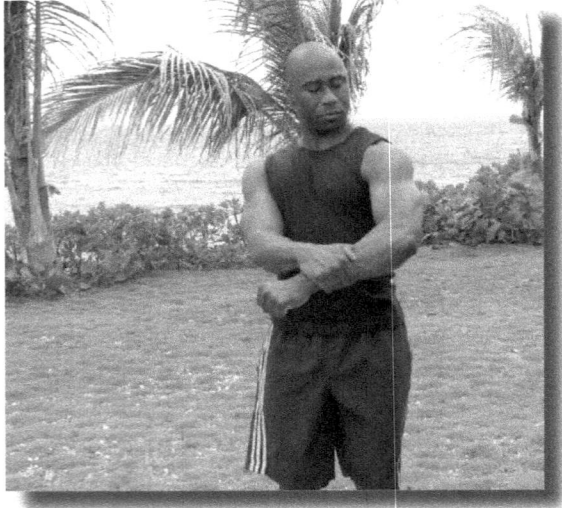

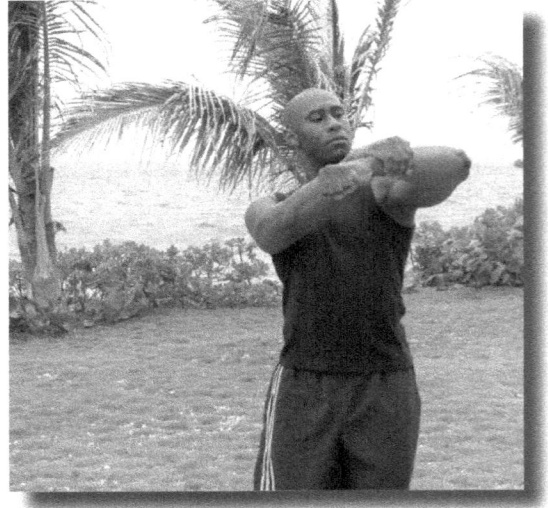

Across the Body Lateral Raises (Stretch and Contracted)

Grasp the left arm that is across the body as in the picture. Now raise the arm outwards towards the side contracted position resisting with the right arm. Perform desired reps then switch arms.

CHAPTER 4

BODYPART ANALYSIS (EXPLANATION)
SHOULDER EXERCISES

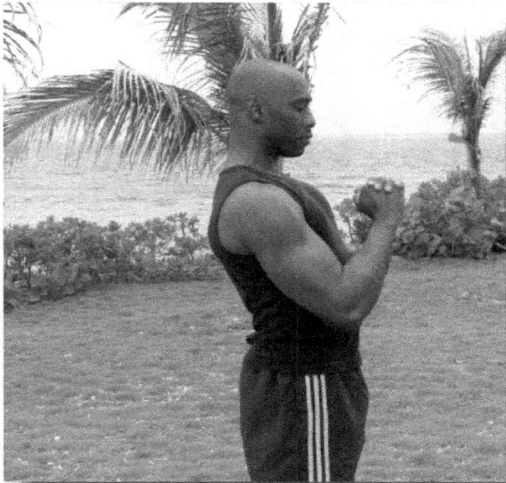

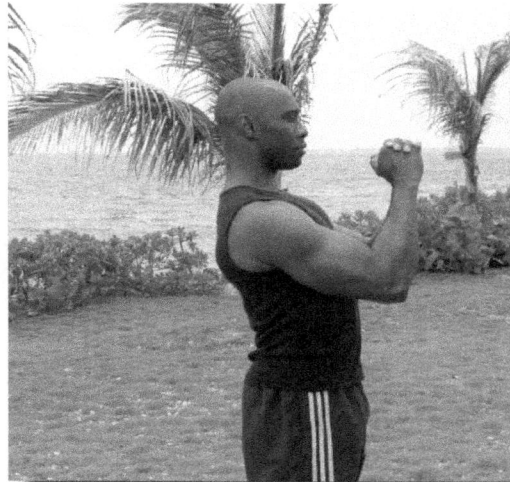

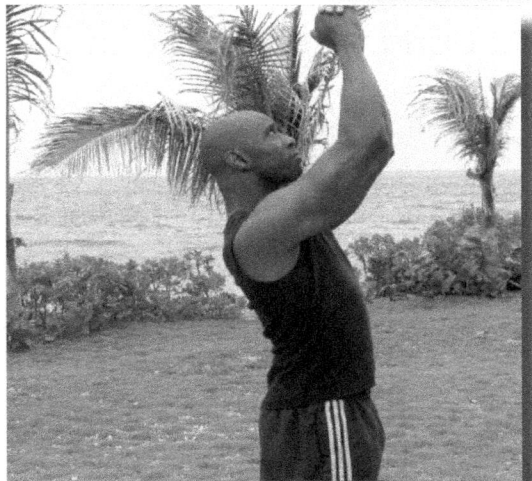

Resisted Shoulder Press (Basic and Contracted)

Place the left hand on-top of the right fist. Press the right arm upwards while resisting with the left hand. Reverse the movement at the top by pulling the left hand downwards while resisting with the right. Continue for reps then switch arms.

CHAPTER 4

BODYPART ANALYSIS (EXPLANATION)
SHOULDER EXERCISES

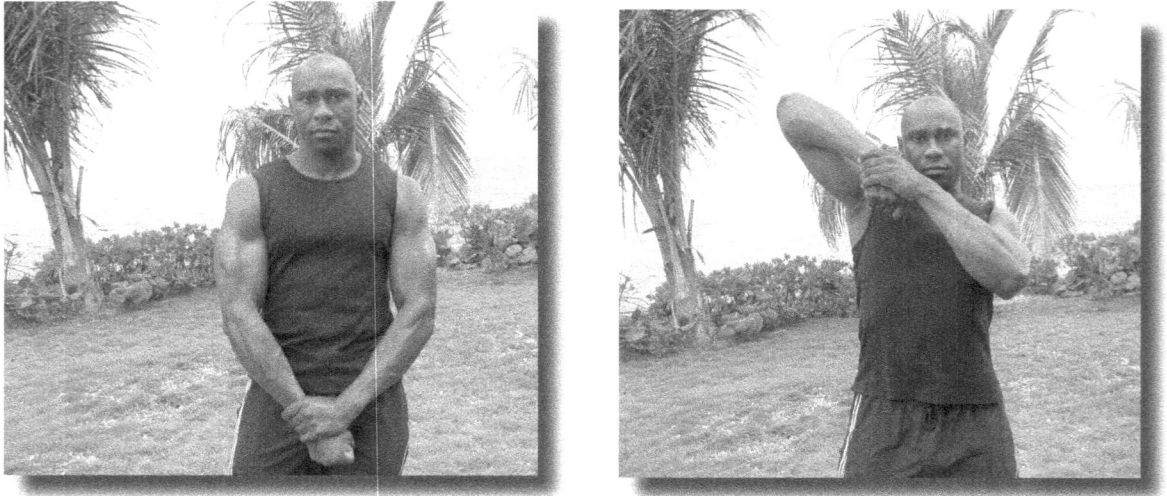

Resisted Upright Pulls (Basic and Contracted)

Hold onto the right wrist as shown above. Now pull the right arm upward while resisting with the left arm. Pull towards the ear, relax and repeat.

CHAPTER 4

BODYPART ANALYSIS (EXPLANATION)
BICEP EXERCISES

Ok I've made a few changes to the original resisted curl to make it far more effective in building strength shape and muscle faster than before. At the very beginning while performing the original resisted curl gains were good but not great. Once I learned how to make the exercise harder and more efficient that's when my biceps and forearms really started to grow and take shape. It's all about efficiency in effort by changing this around to make it work better for you.

People are always looking at anyone that walk up that look a little fit or muscular, and what's the first thing they look at? The biceps and forearms. That's the first thing they see really. I've noticed it and all the people I've talked to about it have said so as well. It also helps when there's veins all around. What I've realized is that while I was developing or trying to develop my biceps and forearms my forearms got wider and was impressive when flexed , but my biceps looked narrow and when flexed flat looking.

My biceps weren't as impressive hanging to my sides. It wasn't wide enough. So I paid attention to the exercises that would make a difference and one of the lessons I learned is to change the way I did the regular Atlas curls at different angles and hand positioning. This made a difference with increasing the diameter of my biceps. Now when I stood, I looked at my biceps in the mirror it's the inner part of the bicep that gives that width!

Height is another thing that the long head on the outside and the muscle that's under the bicep needs to be developed as well..the brachialis. Anyway, lets focus on what I did for the first phase then we'll break things down with the special Bicep and Tricep section later in this mini course. So here we go: Let's look at the muscle Sculpting exercises.

Other than flat abdominals nothing quite says "I'm healthy" than well developed triceps and biceps. Aside from appearance, strong arms can also enhance your athletic performance in any sport your play. Although most people focus on the biceps, developing the triceps is equally important. The following exercises do both.

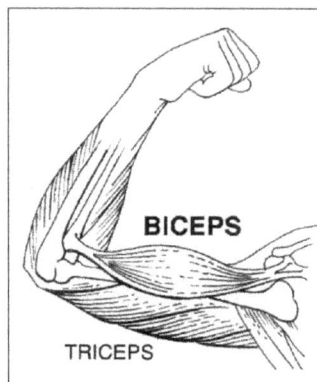

BICEPS

TRICEPS

CHAPTER 4

BODYPART ANALYSIS (EXPLANATION)
BICEP EXERCISES

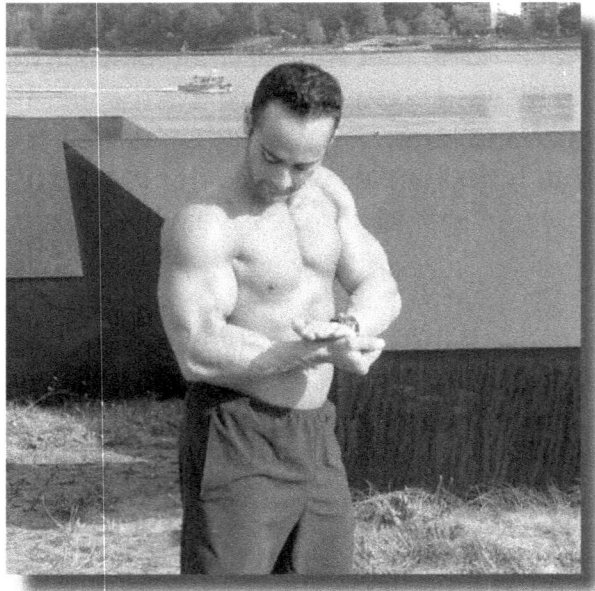

Palm up bicep curls

CHAPTER 4

BODYPART ANALYSIS (EXPLANATION)
BICEP EXERCISES

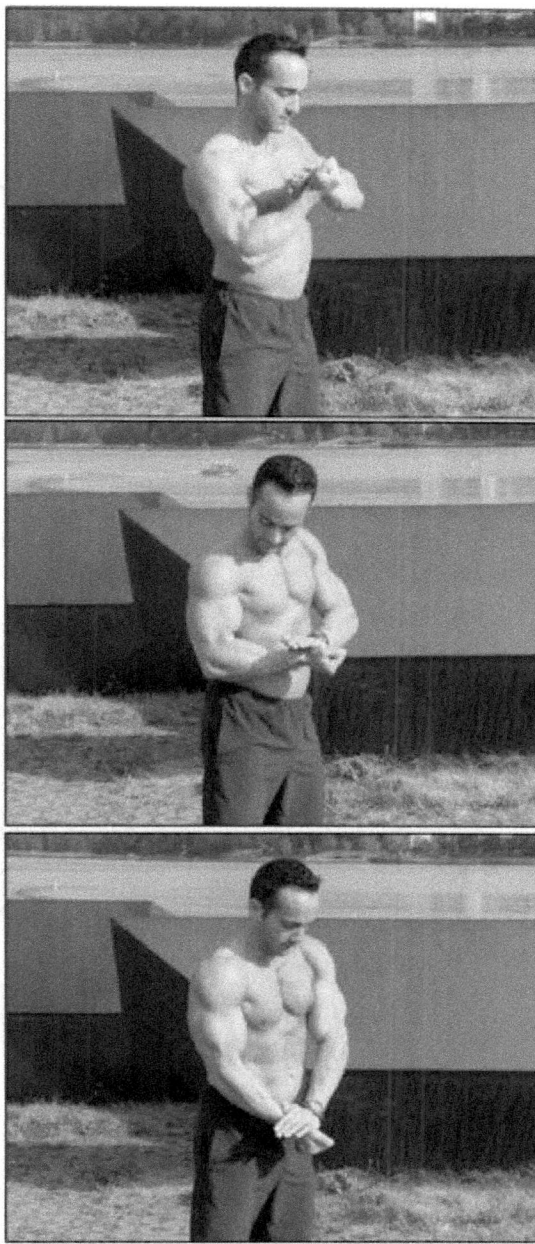

Bicep Curl (Palm Up) (Basic)

Grasp your right fist with the left hand. Pull the right arm upward towards the shoulder while resisting with the left hand. At the shoulder, reverse the exercise by pushing the left arm downwards resisting with the right. Continue for reps then switch arms.

CHAPTER 4

BODYPART ANALYSIS (EXPLANATION)
BICEP/FOREARM EXERCISES

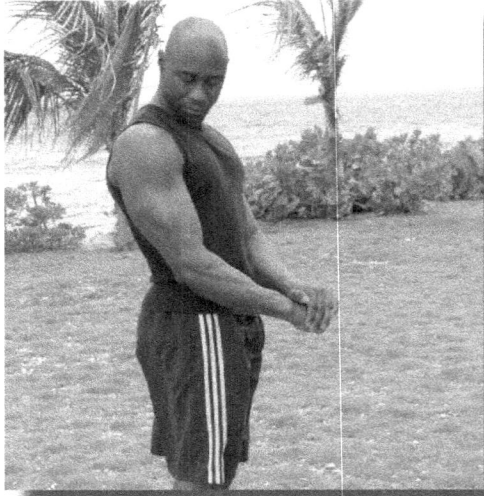

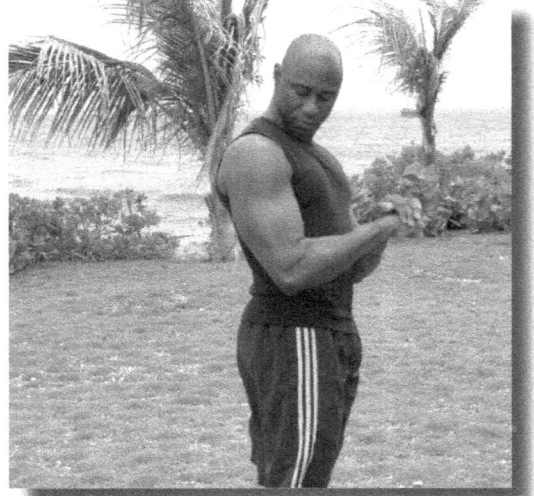

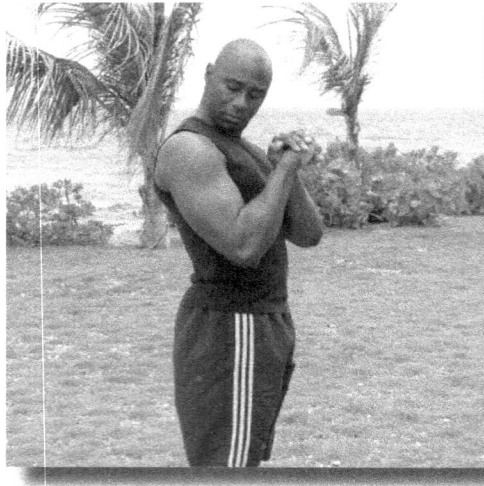

Reverse Bicep/Forearm Curls

This is the Grand-daddy of all exercises. A great bicep/forearm widener. Place the left hand on top of the right fist. Now pull the right hand upwards while resisting with the left hand. At the shoulder reverse the exercise by pushing the left arm downwards resisting with the right hand. Repeat for reps then switch arms.

CHAPTER 4

BODYPART ANALYSIS (EXPLANATION)
BICEP/FOREARM EXERCISES

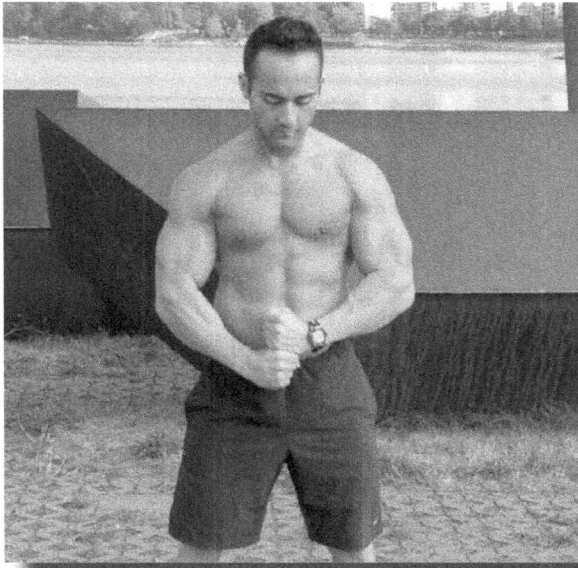

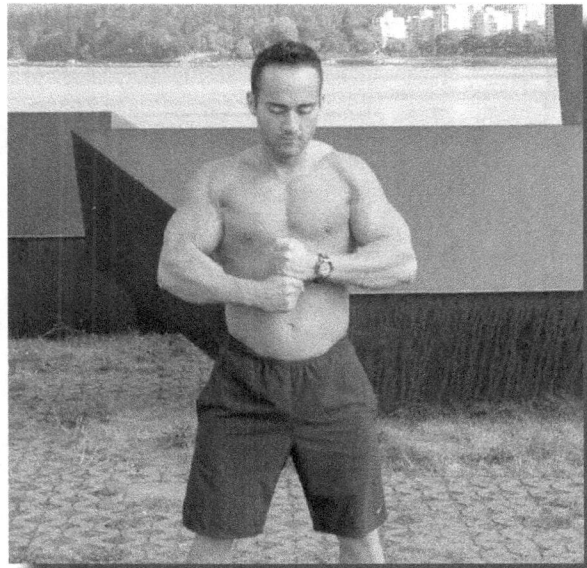

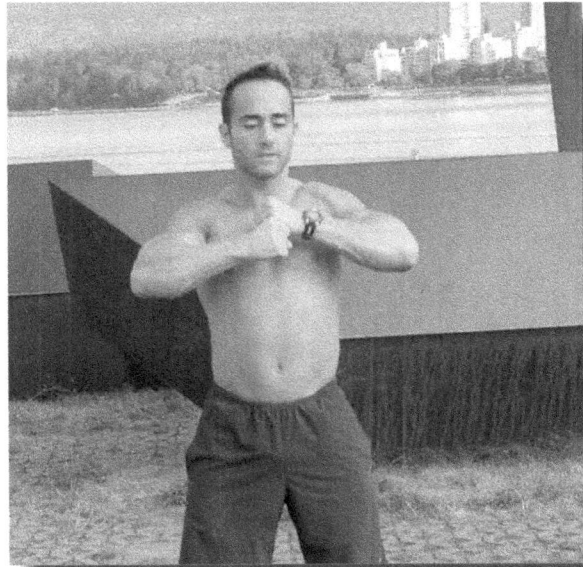

Hammer Curls

Another great Bicep/Forearm combo. Place the wrists as shown in the picture above. Now pull with the right hand or bottom hand upwards to the chest while resisting with the top hand. At upper chest level reverse the exercise by pressing the top wrist down and resisting with the bottom wrist. Repeat for reps then switch arms.

CHAPTER 4

BODYPART ANALYSIS (EXPLANATION)
BICEP/FOREARM EXERCISES

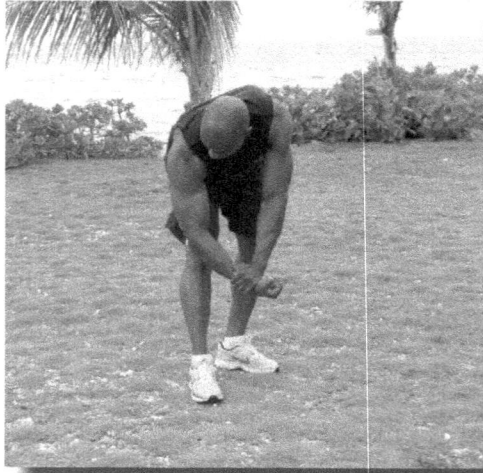

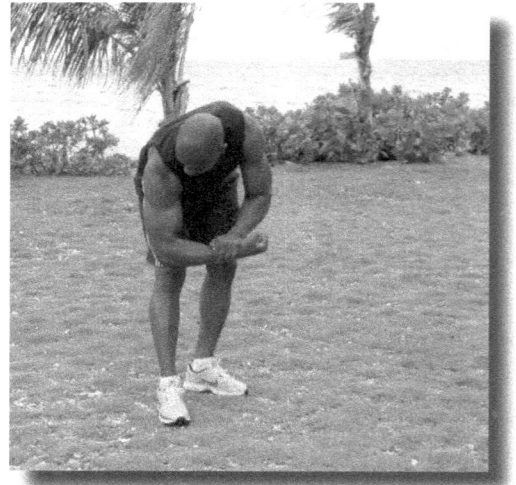

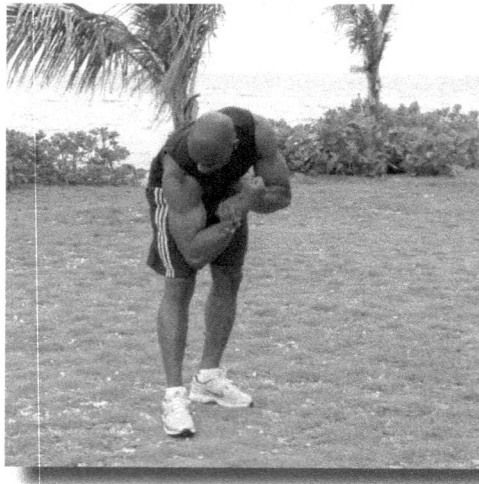

Concentration Curls (contracted)

This is a great bicep finisher move. Peak contraction to hit that long head again. As pictured in start position hold onto the right wrist with left hand and pull the right arm towards the face while resisting with the left hand. Now reverse the exercise by pushing the left arm down and resisting with the right. Complete your reps then switch arms and repeat movement.

CHAPTER 4

BODYPART ANALYSIS (EXPLANATION)
TRICEP EXERCISES

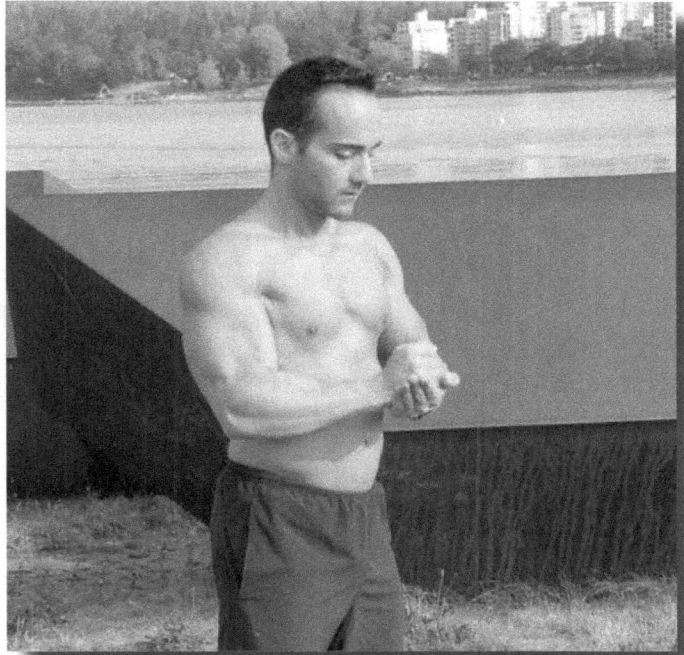

Tricep pressdown

CHAPTER 4

BODYPART ANALYSIS (EXPLANATION)
TRICEP EXERCISES

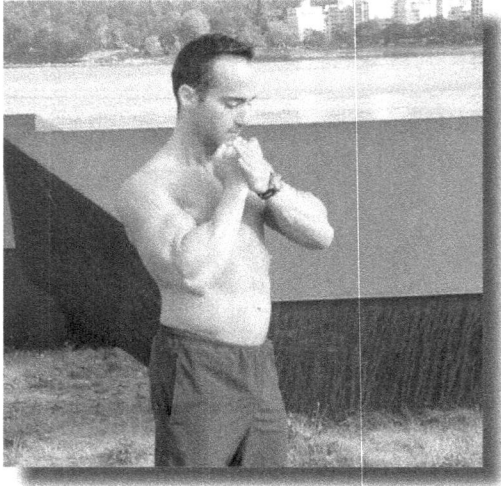

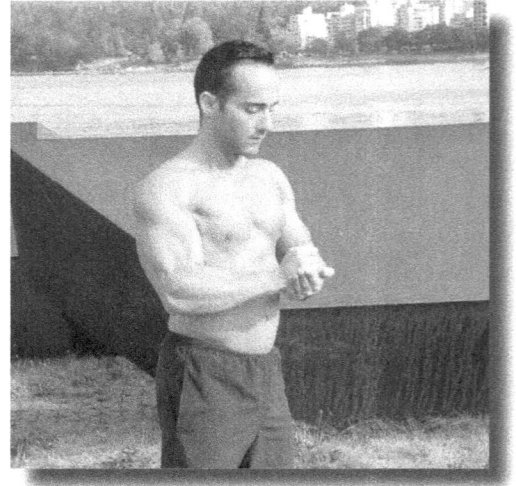

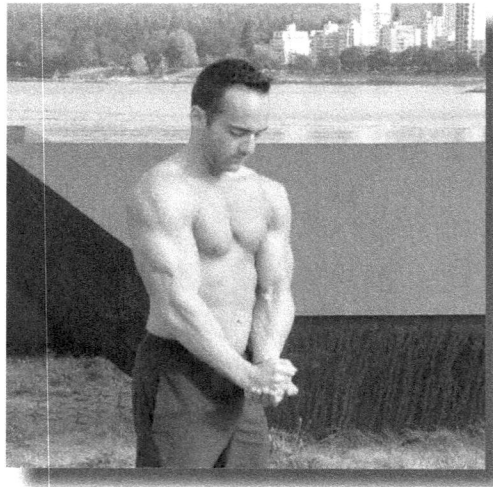

Tricep pressdown

The triceps long head is the largest part of the tricep musculature. It's responsible for the most tricep size. The tricep is broken into 3 muscle-heads. Lateral (outer head), Long Head (inside muscle), and the Middle or medial head. (middle muscle). The tricep is easily developed due to dips, pushups and a variety of self resistance type exercises. The self resistance exercises are geared to stimulate the tricep throughout the full range motion through 3 separate ranges of push.

CHAPTER 4

BODYPART ANALYSIS (EXPLANATION)
TRICEP EXERCISES

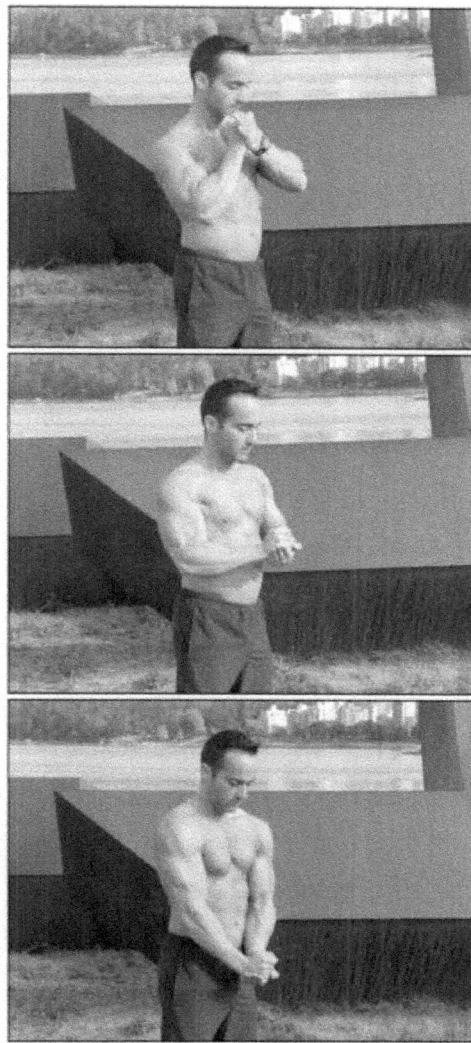

Tricep pressdown

Make a fist with the right hand and place it in the left. Now press the right hand downwards while resisting with the left hand. Repeat desired reps then switch arms.

CHAPTER 4

BODYPART ANALYSIS (EXPLANATION)
TRICEP EXERCISES

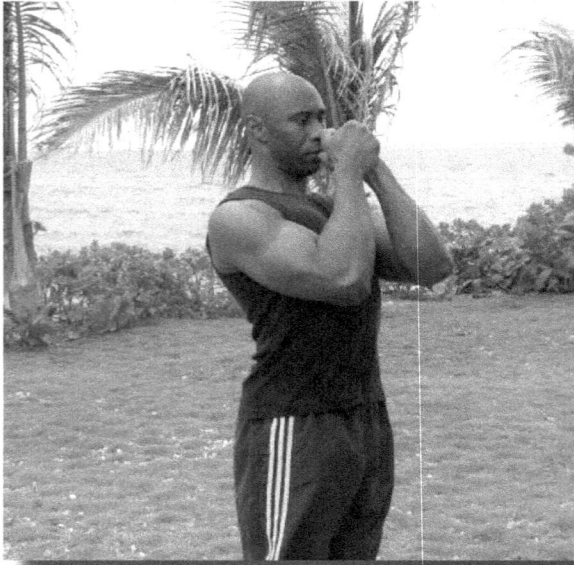

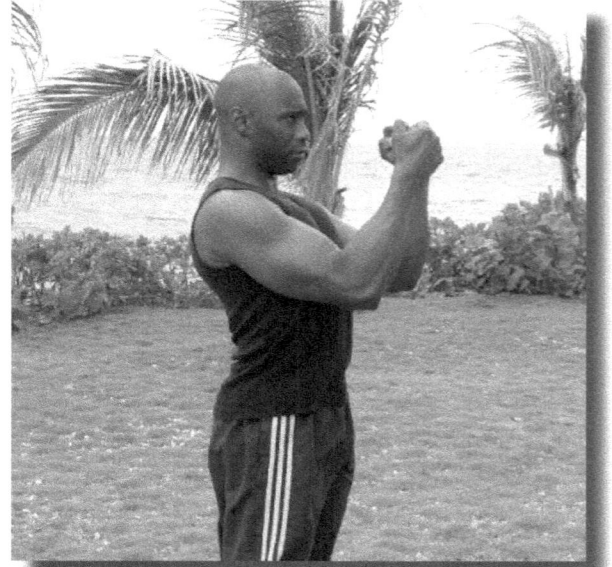

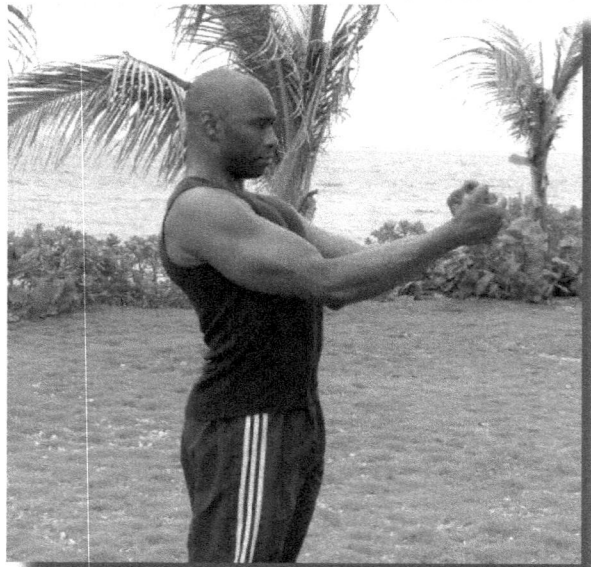

Forward Lateral Press (Basic)

Place the left fist in the right hand. Now push the left hand forward while resisting with the right hand. At the finished position reverse the movement by pulling the right hand towards you resisting with the left.

CHAPTER 4

BODYPART ANALYSIS (EXPLANATION)
TRICEP EXERCISES

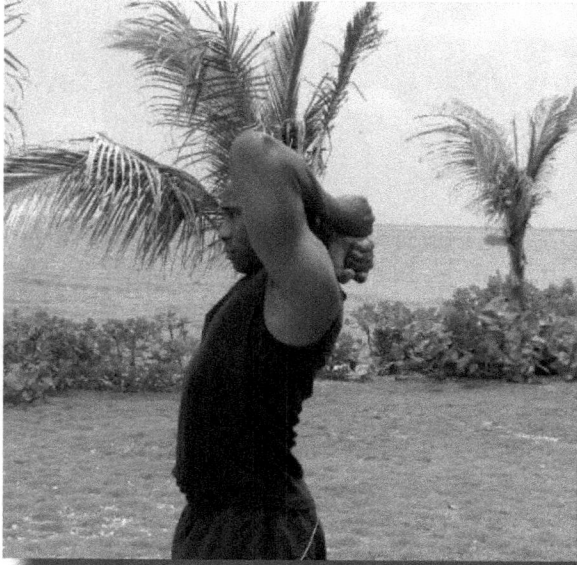

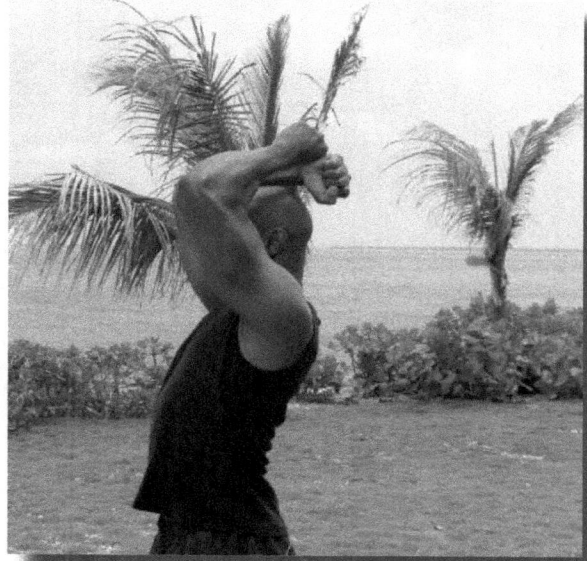

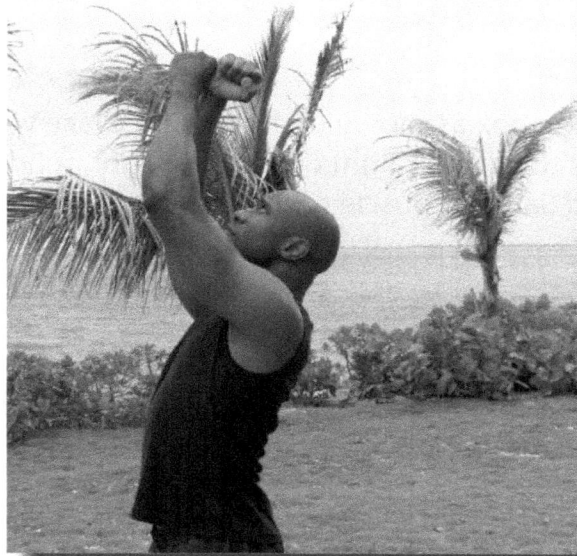

Over Head Tricep Press (stretch, contracted)

Make a fist with both hands place it behind your neck. Now press the bottom fist upward while resisting with the top fist. At the top reverse the exercise by pushing downwards with the top fist while resisting with the bottom fist. Use a light to moderate tension due to the tricep tendons being quite sensitive at that position.

CHAPTER 4

BODYPART ANALYSIS (EXPLANATION)
TRICEP EXERCISES

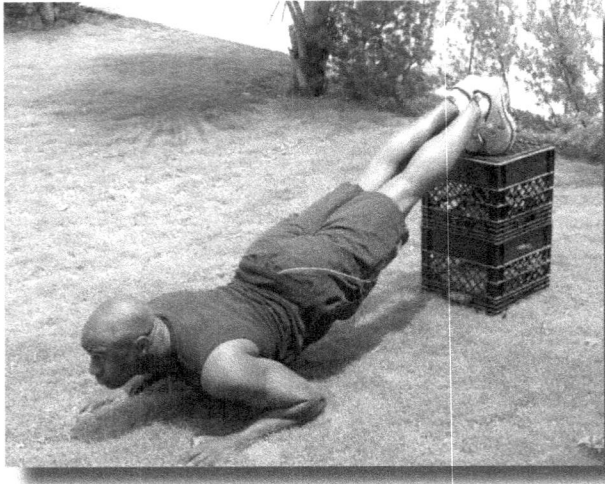

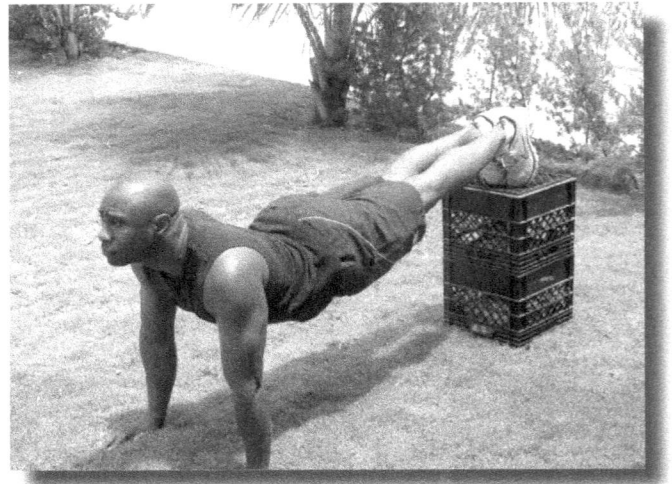

Decline Tricep Extensions (Basic)

Place your feet on a chair or box as shown in the picture. Place your hands and lower-arms on the floor and slowly press the arm straight out with a slight bend to the elbows. This exercise stimulates the outer head (lateral) muscle of the triceps.

CHAPTER 4

BODYPART ANALYSIS (EXPLANATION)
FOREARM EXERCISES

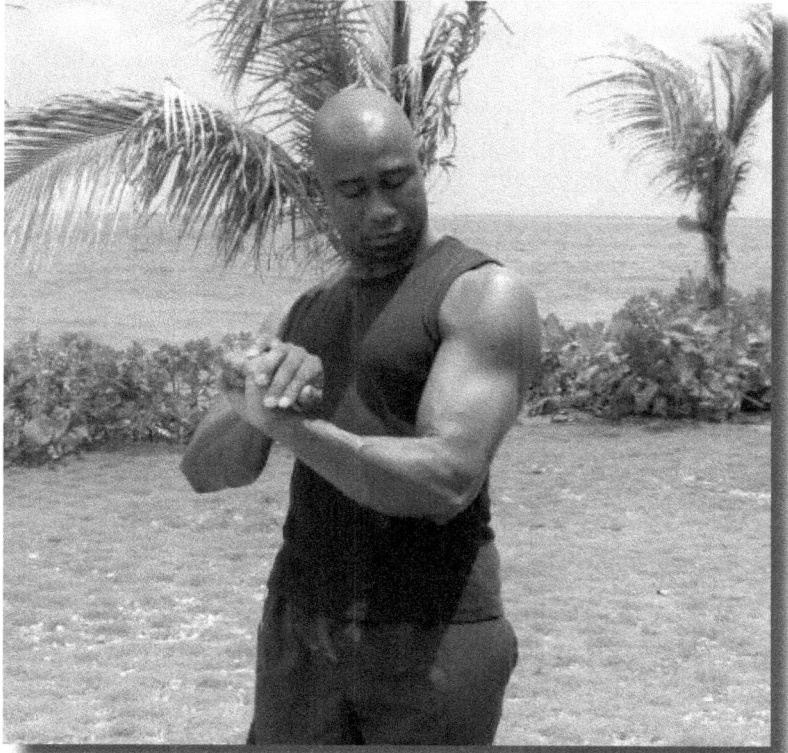

Wrist curls palm down

Powerful forearms just like upper arms command respect! This muscle needs to be balanced with the upper arm. Last thing you want are forearms that look weak with powerful upper-arms. So, here's a number of exercises to increase the griping strength, and overall muscula-ture of the lower arm, connective tissues of the wrists and increases and strengthens the grip.

CHAPTER 4

BODYPART ANALYSIS (EXPLANATION)
FOREARM EXERCISES

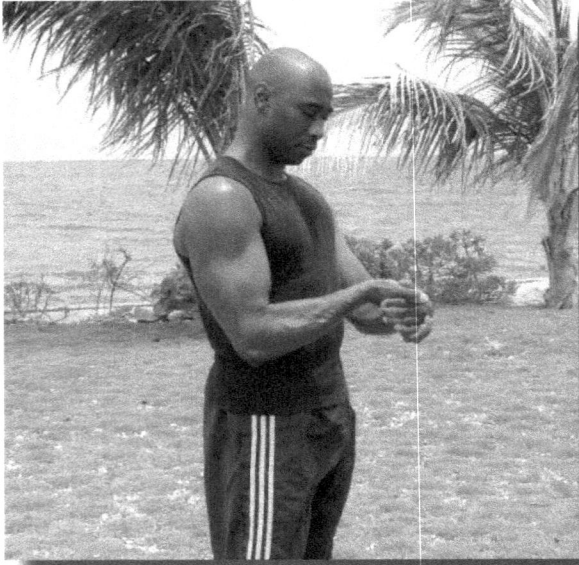

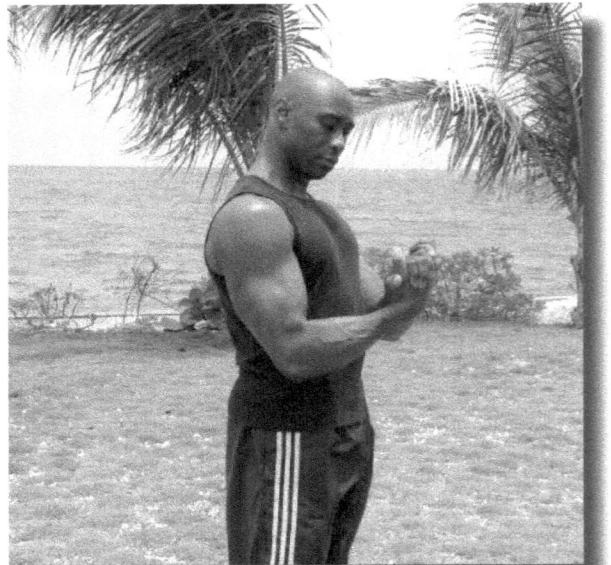

Palm Up Wrist Curls

As pictured extend the right wrist backwards placing the left hand pressed against. Now Flex the right wrist upwards while resisting with the left hand. Practice till tired or desired reps are done then switch hands and repeat.

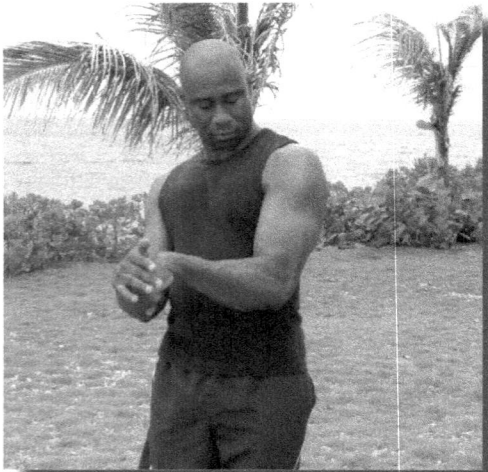

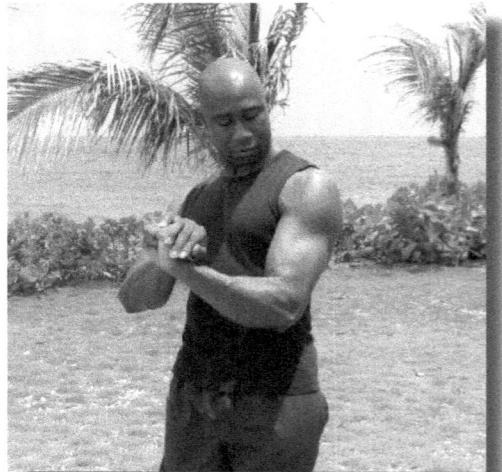

Same as before but this time the palm in pressed down. Resist with the opposite hand for reps then reverse hands.

CHAPTER 4

BODYPART ANALYSIS (EXPLANATION)
FOREARM EXERCISES

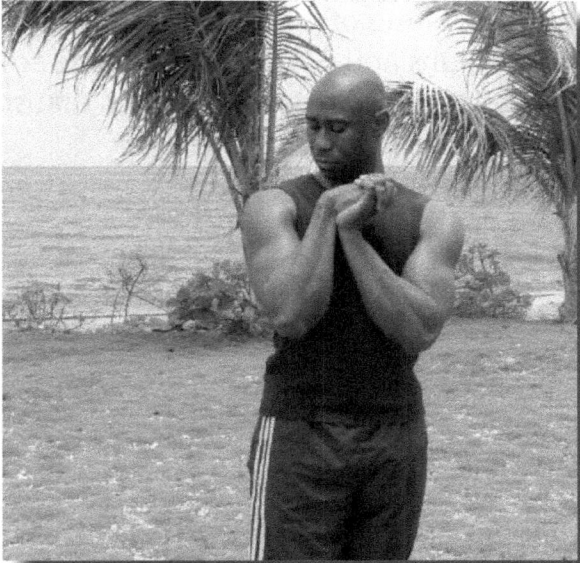

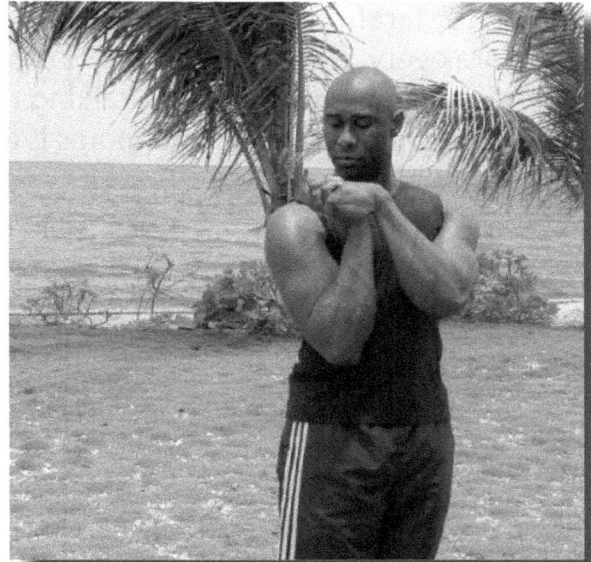

Forearm presses

Perform this exercise as pictured by pressing to one side then the other while resisting with the opposite hand.

CHAPTER 4

BODYPART ANALYSIS (EXPLANATION) THIGH AND HAMSTRING EXERCISES

Ok let's focus on the Powerful thighs and hamstring development exercises. Developing strength and power is what every athlete as well as every person wants. How do we achieve that? Let's start from the very top: One Legged Squats the King of All Lower-Body exercises stimulate everything! Thighs, Hips, Hamstrings, Inner Thighs and Glutes (butt). Followed by Leg extensions, and leg curls we are talking maximum efficiency. Multi-Joint exercises that stimulate the important hips, thighs and glutes is all we need. Let's get on with it..

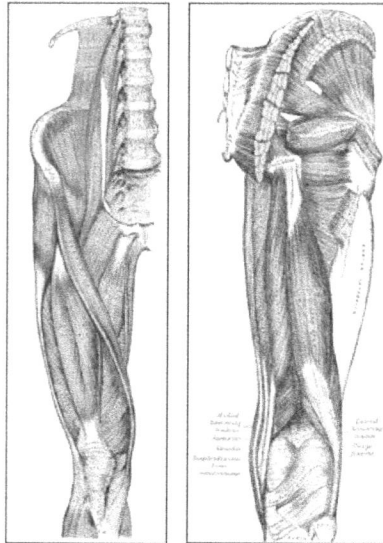

The hip and thigh muscles are the largest in the body. Athletic, muscular legs are not only attractive and vital to playing sports, but they are also one of the keys to staying young. "Healthy legs act like a heart for the lower body", someone once said, and they're right. If you want to stay young, you need to keep that blood pumping. Healthy legs will keep you young, strong and vital for life.

CHAPTER 4

BODYPART ANALYSIS (EXPLANATION)
THIGH AND HAMSTRING EXERCISES

Few exercises are as impressive as a properly conducted one-leg-squat. Some of the best athletes and strength coaches in the world are unable to perfrom a single rep of this advanced exercise, let alone a full set of them. In time, though, with solid practice you will develop an awesome pair of muscular thighs, hmstrings and inner thighs to go along with it.

Stand with your knees slightly bent and your arms outstretched to balance. Lift one leg off the ground and place it as far out in front of you as possible while keeping it straight. (don't worry you will get better in time). Then, slowly lower yourself as far as possible on your balancing leg. When your hamstrings touch your calves (or as far as you can perform this exercise at first), push back up with the supporting leg to the start possition and repeat.

If your balance isn't tip top perform the exercise holding onto a chair with a free hand for support.

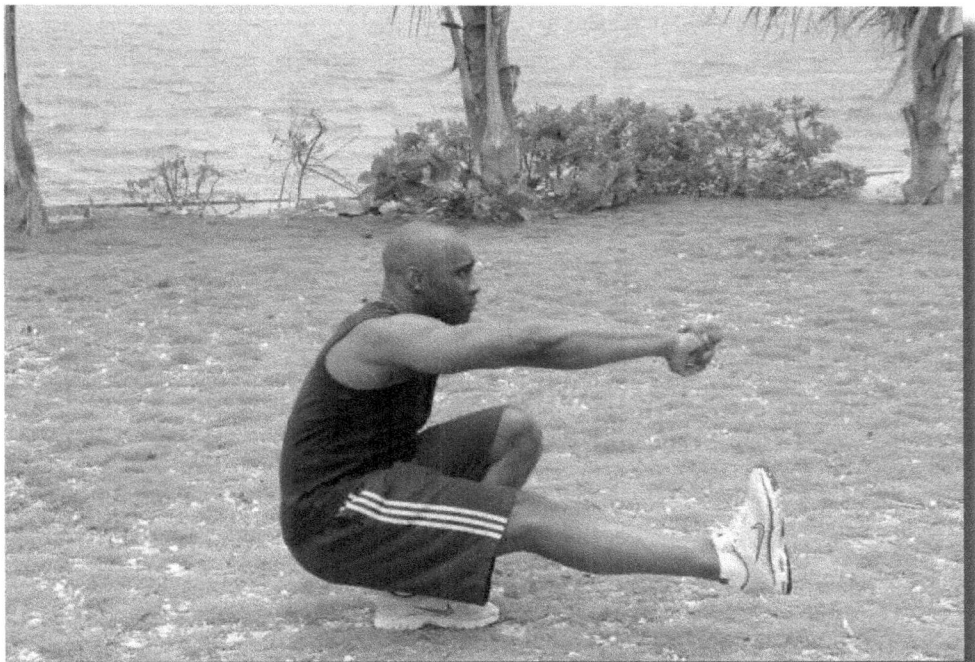

One Legged Squats

CHAPTER 4

BODYPART ANALYSIS (EXPLANATION)
THIGH AND HAMSTRING EXERCISES

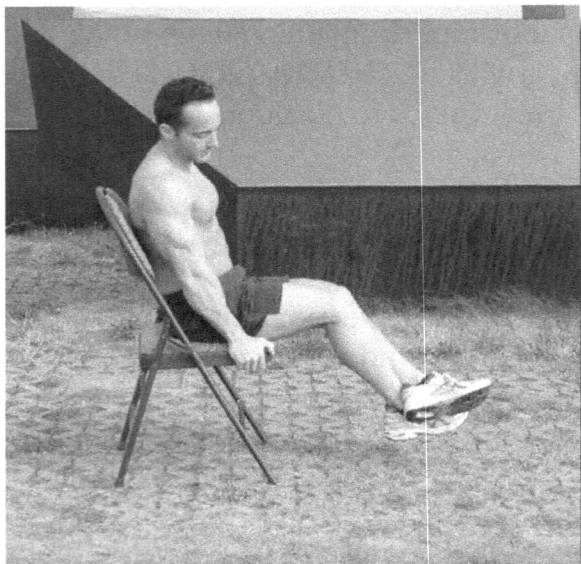

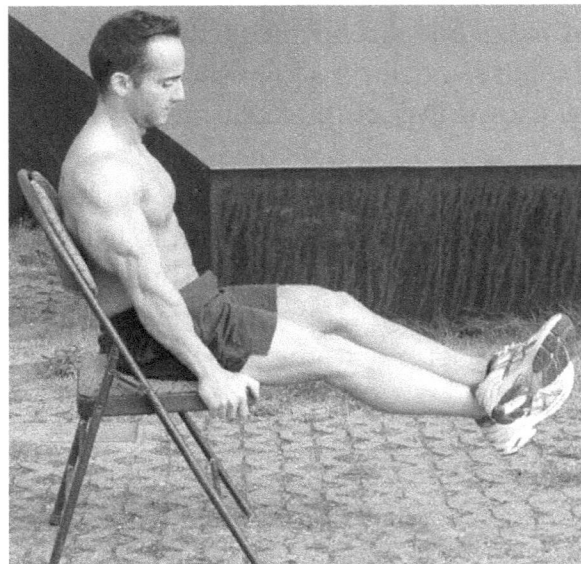

Resisted Leg Extensions

While seated on a chair, box or stool, place the right leg over the left as shown in the picture, and extend the left leg outwards resisting with the right. At the top reverse the movement by pulling down the right while resisting with the left.

CHAPTER 4

BODYPART ANALYSIS (EXPLANATION)
THIGH AND HAMSTRING EXERCISES

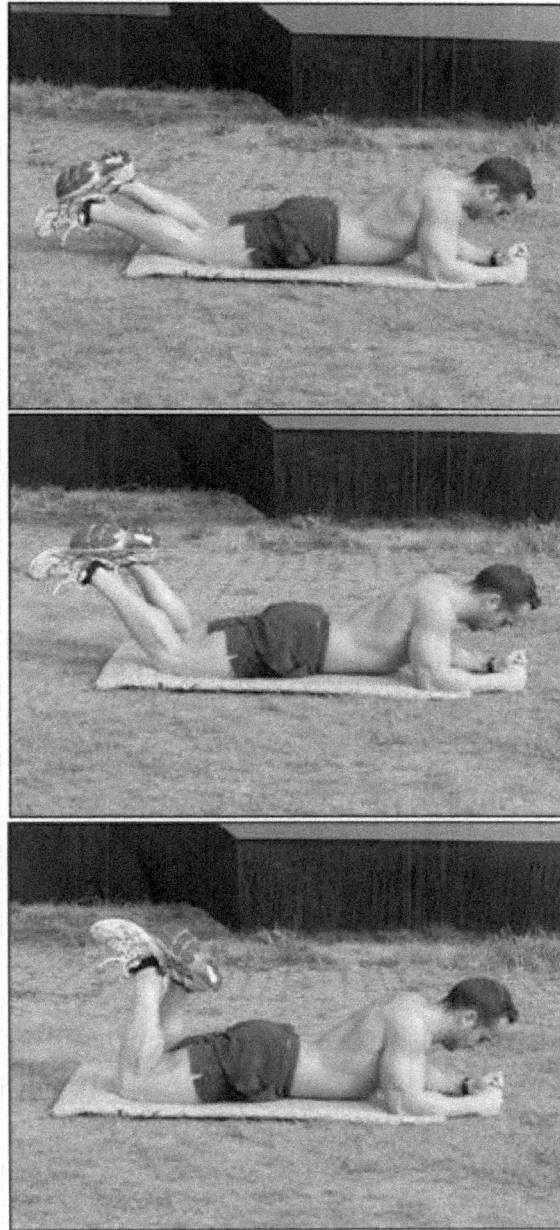

Hamstring Resisted Leg Curl

While on the stomach on the floor place the left leg over the right as shown, Now pull the right leg upwards towards you while resisting with the left leg. Pull on the Up phase only. Repeat for reps then switch legs.

CHAPTER 4

BODYPART ANALYSIS (EXPLANATION)
CALVE EXERCISES

Now calf growth due to the dense layers of the muscles itself is quite stubborn! So my results within this department wasn't the best. However, I've learned a few things. In order for my calves to improve various steps had to be taken into consideration. I did loads of high reps daily but lost the true meaning of building muscle within this area. In order to add muscle onto those it's best to really focus on how you're doing the exercises and what rep range you're using for ultimate muscle building stimulation, which I'll explain in a moment). Here they are:

Stretch: You achieve this position at the bottom of any calf exercise—calves stretched off a high block. It's important to get that stretch to force the calves to contract at it's maximum!

HIGH REPS. As I've said earlier the calve is one dense muscle. The majority of these calf fibers are Endurance Oriented Fibers. Because it's used daily. You contract these muscles all day by walking. So they need to be taxed a certain way. The best way to target the calves are with reps that hit the range between 30 to 35 reps per set. Tension times are increased for your straight sets of calf work and should be about one minute or more, to efficiently hit the dense fibers effectively.

FEEL. As with any muscle group you must pay attention to the feel and focus on the muscle at hand. It is important to avoid bouncing and fast reps. Rep speed is also important.
Three seconds up and the same speed for the down portion is about right. But feel is the most important element here. Another key to maximizing calf development and to increase the stress is to maintain the tension on the calve muscles.

By not coming all the way up to full contraction this maintains constant tension on the muscle and increases blood blockage. This will indeed increase growth stimulation, capillary development and muscle overload and what about the bottom range? This is just as important.
It's important to get a max stretch at the bottom of the movement. This really pre-stretches the muscles to fire more efficiently due to the powerful stretch that loosens up the fibers, which produces additional growth.

CHAPTER 4

BODYPART ANALYSIS (EXPLANATION)
CALVE EXERCISES

More Calf-Growing Details

Now guys I don't have genetically superior calve development. Well not yet anyway..still working on it. After my experiment I added a component that was never done for my calves effectively, but last year my calves got even better than the year before with less work per set. They looked almost two inches bigger. It didn't make sense really. So I introduced a number of techniques and stress methods into my calve workouts for the first time.

To see the effects of it all. Lo and behold my calves responded far better to the stress methods. After all, my calves looked much better with more size and shape and increased vascularity more naturally. Now I'm not blessed with inner-calf flare. So seeing that the methods increased that fact I loved it to the max! By doubling up on the key contracted point of the movement with mini reps at the end of my full reps made the set far more intense. That's only one method I did. You will see more in later chapters in the routine sections.

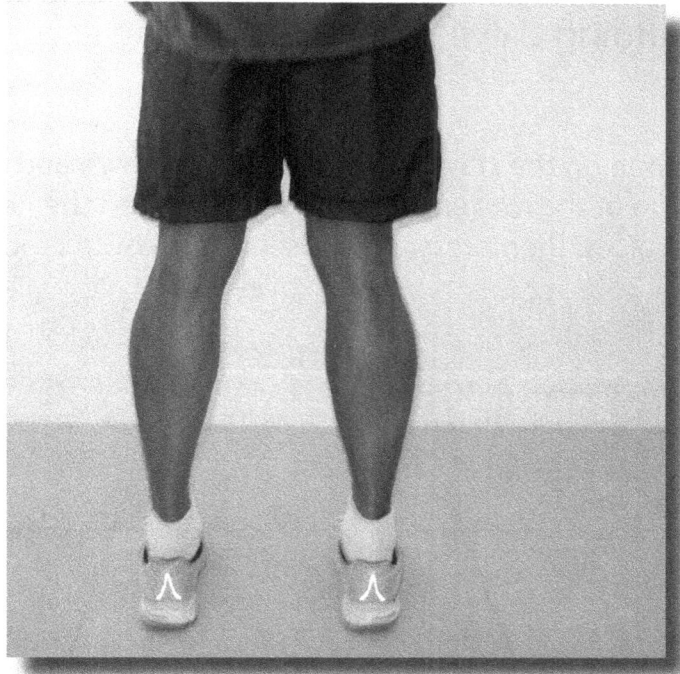

CHAPTER 4

BODYPART ANALYSIS (EXPLANATION)
CALVE EXERCISES

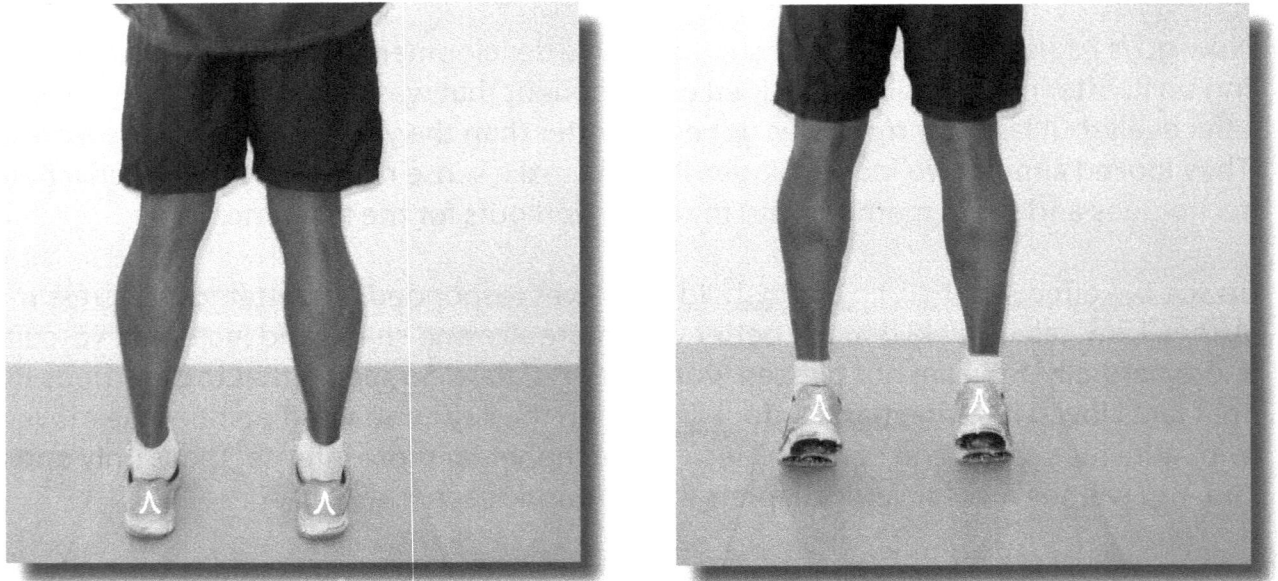

Standing Calve Raises (stretch and contracted)

This exercise can be done on the stairs or block. Start as shown and go up and down contracting the calves at the top of the movement. If on stairs, extend the heels as low as you can to really pre-stretch the calves, then press upwards into the contracted position.

CHAPTER 4

BODYPART ANALYSIS (EXPLANATION)
CALVE EXERCISES

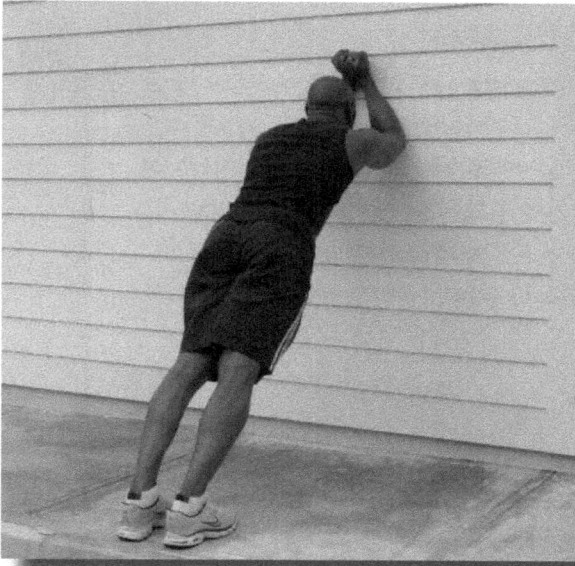

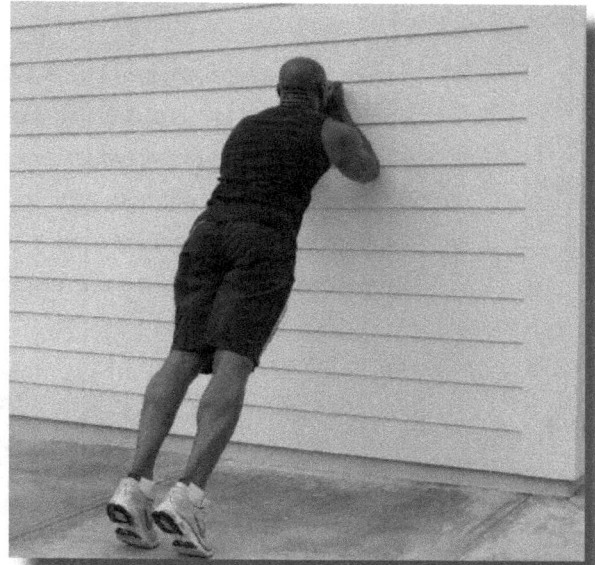

Slanted Pre-Stretch Calve Raises

Stand at least 30 inches away from the wall, or position yourself as shown but make sure the calves are well stretched. Start off as shown in the picture start position. Press straight up on the toes then lower. This is as awesome calve stretch exercise. Perform this exercise until the calves are well tired. This stimulates the entire calve.

CHAPTER 4

BODYPART ANALYSIS (EXPLANATION) ABDOMINAL EXERCISES

For aesthetics everyone wants a flat stomach and a six-pack abs look. However, there's more to the abdominal than just looks. Strong abdominal muscles will not only help you maintain youthfulness and vigor but will enhance the functionality of every gland and organ in your trunk. They also aid in digestion and elimination. Note that if you want the 6 pack abs look you will need to watch your body fat level. For men this usually means less than 10% body fat and for women less than 14%.

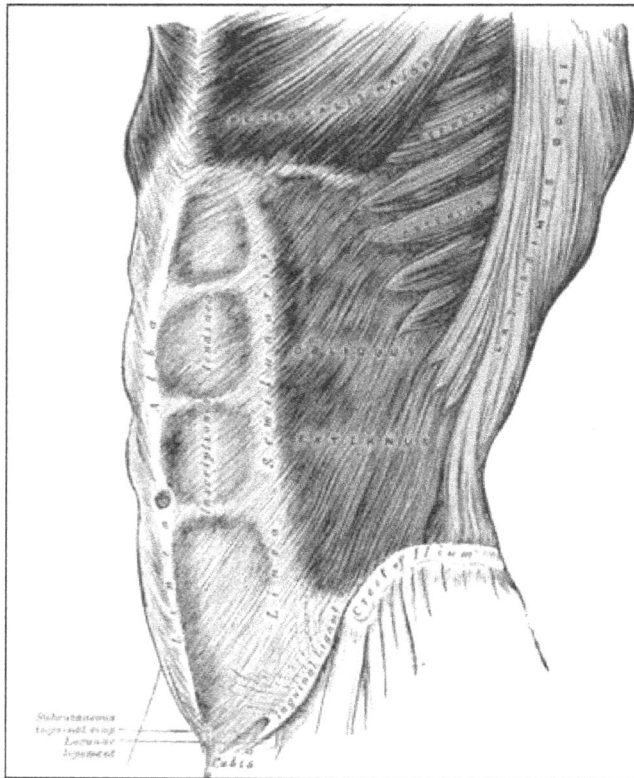

CHAPTER 4

BODYPART ANALYSIS (EXPLANATION) ABDOMINAL EXERCISES

Abdominal Training are endurance type fiber muscles. Very much like forearms and calve muscles. Which means they need longer tension times and high rep ranges to benefit from training.

Muscle Makeup: The abdominal muscles are just that—muscles. It's one sheet of muscles with tendons dividing the muscles into blocks. So, it isn't upper and lower it's one sheet. Each is made up of the same types of fibers as your biceps, chest and back; however, as I mentioned, many of the fibers in the abs are more endurance oriented and require higher reps to reach full development.

The main abdominal muscle that one need to be concerned with, is the rectus abdominis, (front area) this isn't a bunch of knotted musles, as it appears to be, but rather a sheet-type muscle that runs from the bottom of your rib cage and attaches to your pelvis. As I've said earlier, the ripples are actually caused by tendons running horizontally and vertically. Throughout the entire length that cause the block type muscle separation you see.

Hip Flexor Function: The hip flexors come into play on many ab exercises, such as reverse crunches. As you'll soon see, the hip flexors are important contributors, when you exercise the rectus abdominis. Upper and lower separation. Like I said, there's no real separation on upper and lower abs.

Studies indicate that the upper rectus abdominis can work somewhat independently of the lower part of the muscle, as it does when you perform crunches. Or abdominal situps (feet extended not anchored) But when you work the lower portion, your upper rectus always comes into play, as in reverse crunches or across the body crunches.

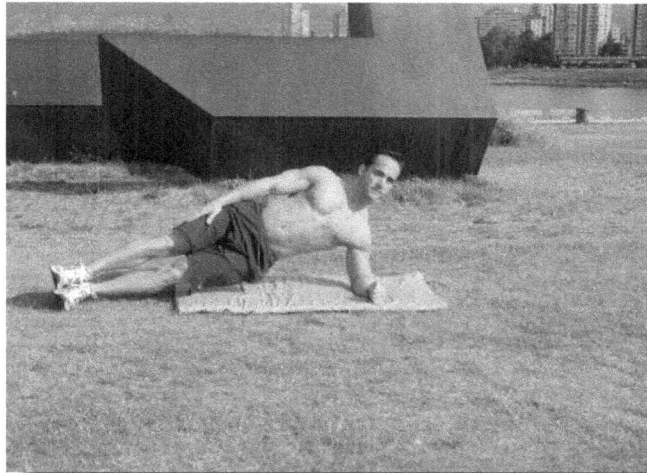

CHAPTER 4

BODYPART ANALYSIS (EXPLANATION)
ABDOMINAL EXERCISES

Therefore, you should always work the lower area first, which brings both upper and lower sections into play. If you isolate the upper part first, you fatigue that area and make your lower-ab work much less effective—in much the same way that working forearms before biceps can limit your biceps efforts. For example, if you do crunches first and then reverse crunches, which works your upper rectus will be so fatigued from the crunches that it'll cause you to fail on the Reverse Crunches long before you fatigue your lower abs—it's one reason so many trainees lack lower-ab delineation:
They work lower abs last or do only crunches in their ab program. So here's just a few exercises that gets the job done. It works the muscles in union in order to get the best of both worlds.

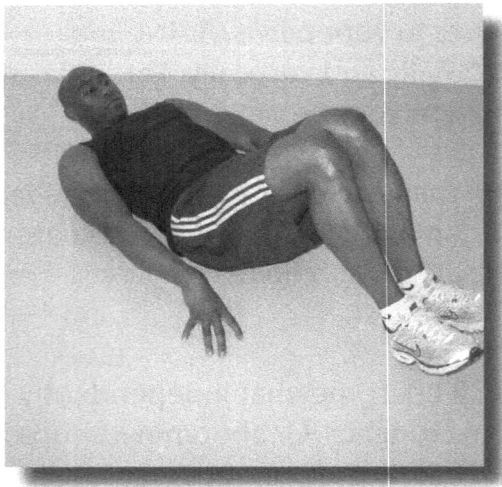

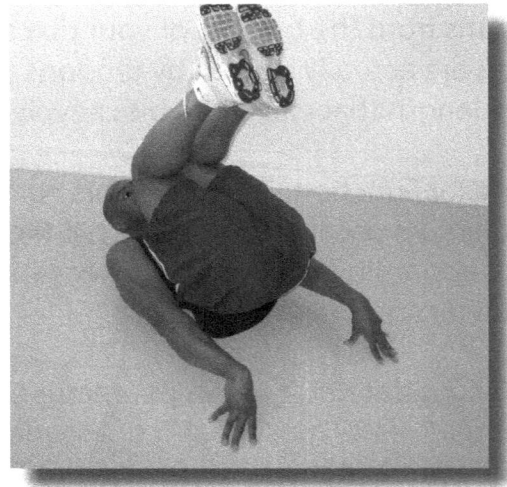

Reverse Crunches

Start as shown in the start position picture. Then roll the hip as you bring the knees into the chest and continue for desired reps.

CHAPTER 4

BODYPART ANALYSIS (EXPLANATION)
ABDOMINAL EXERCISES

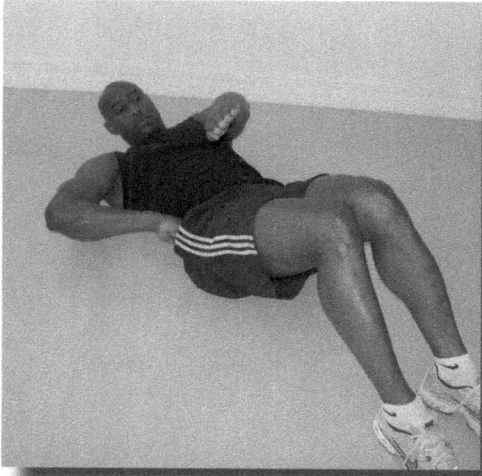

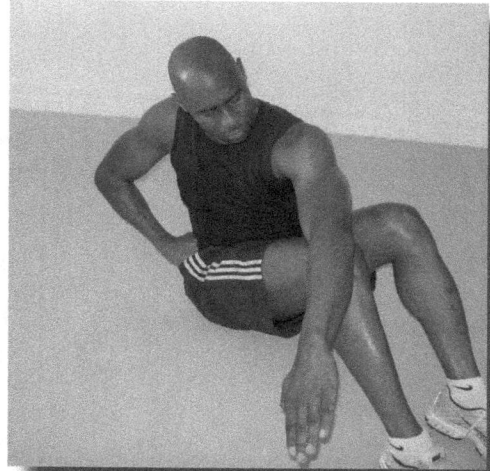

Across-The-Body Situps

Start as shown in first picture. Now raise the upper body upwards and extend the left arm across the right knee as shown. This is a fine exercise for the entire abdominal wall as well as the obliques. After working one side for reps continue with the other in the same manner.

CHAPTER 4

BODYPART ANALYSIS (EXPLANATION)
ABDOMINAL EXERCISES

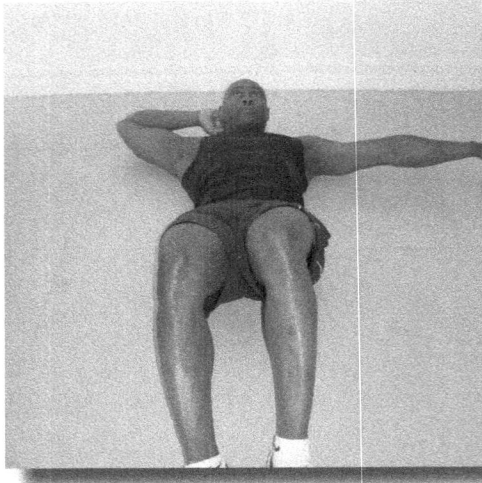
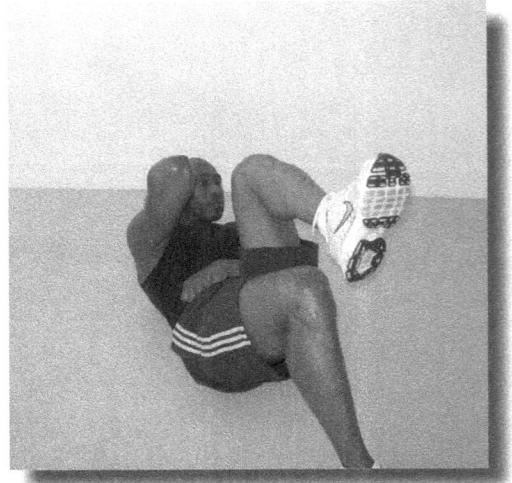

Across-The-Body Side Crunches

Start off flat on the floor with right hand by the ear or behind the head, knees together feet on floor, place the non-working arm on the floor or on the stomach. Now, rotate towards the left knee as shown while bringing it towards the elbow. While touching reverse the movement by going down and lowering the foot in line with the other leg. Perform for reps then change sides.

Another Version

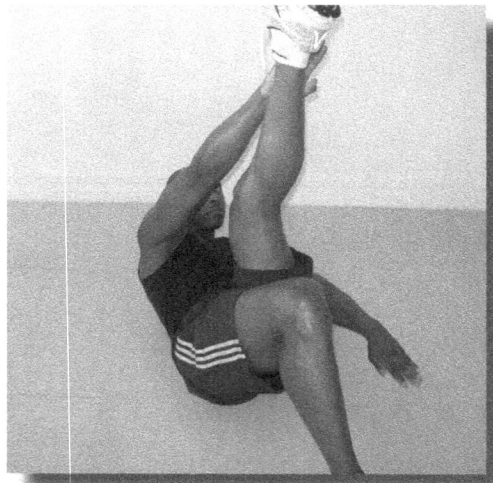

CHAPTER 4

BODYPART ANALYSIS (EXPLANATION)
HAMSTRING/LOWERBACK EXERCISES

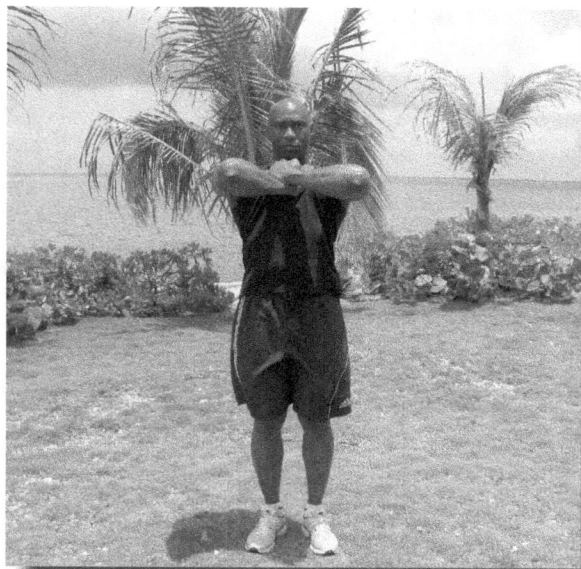

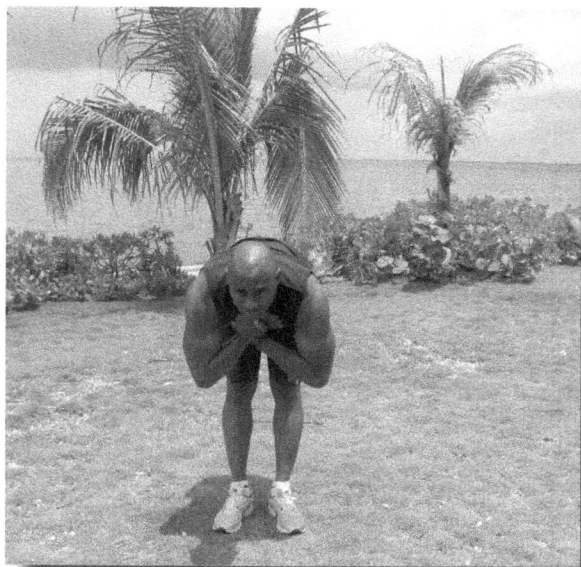

Stiff Legged Presses

Place the hands on your chest. Now, press downwards while resisting with the hands until you are in the finished position. Relax and repeat for reps. This prestretches the hamstrings and adds strength to the lower back musculature.

CHAPTER 4

BODYPART ANALYSIS (EXPLANATION)
THIGH EXERCISES

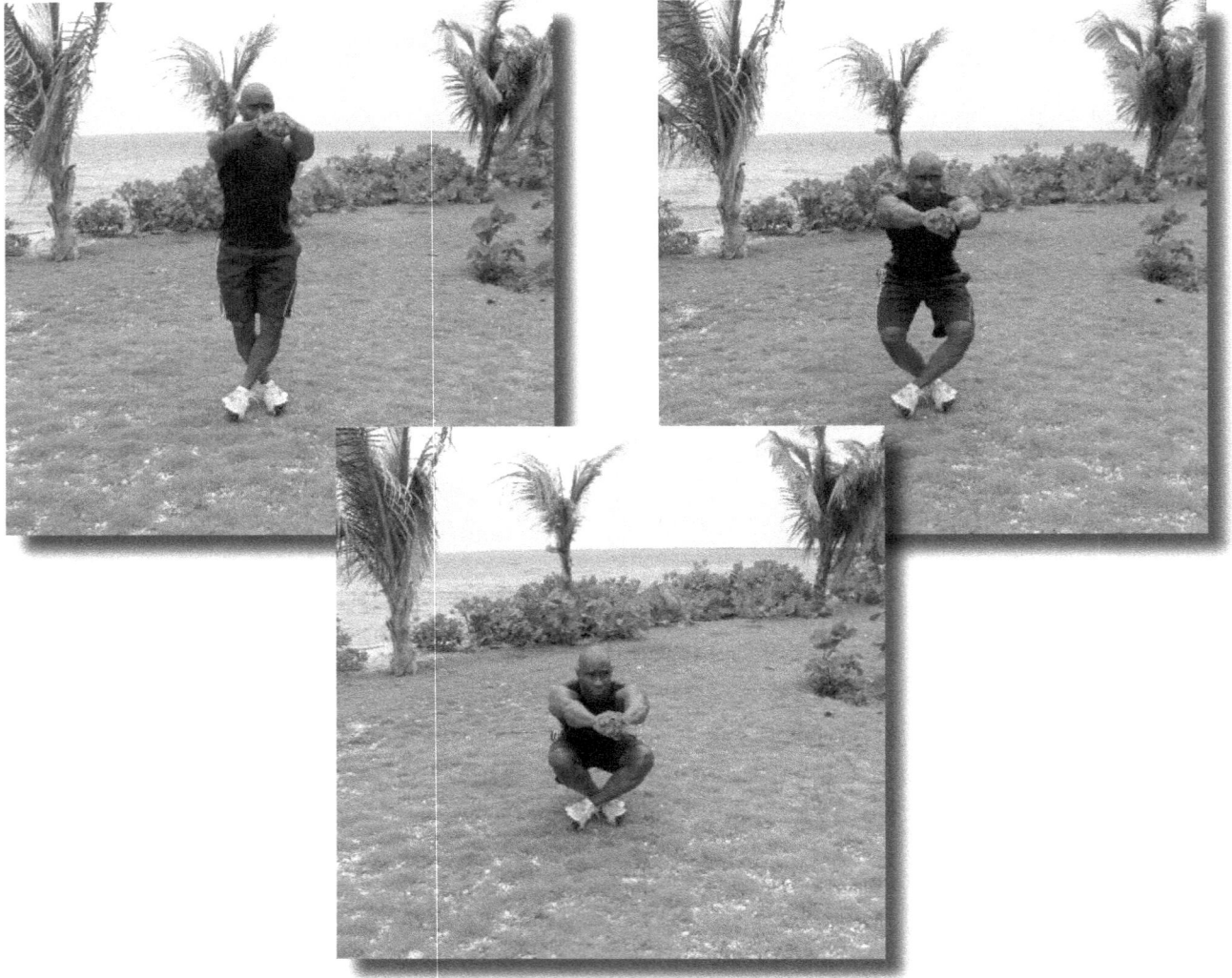

Crossed Feet Squats

Another excellent exercise for the overall thigh and hamstrings. Start off as shown in the starting position with feet crossed. Slowly under control lower yourself to the finished position No Bouncing. One second pause then reverse the movement to the starting position. This exercise may be difficult at first but keep practicing and as night follows day it gets easier.

CHAPTER 5

Phase One (Updated version)

Day One

CHEST
Basic/stretch: Decline pushups (elbows in), 3 sets... 12-15 reps

BACK
Basic: Thigh rows, 3 sets.... 10-12 reps
Basic/stretch: Three chair dips, 3 sets.... 12-15 reps

THIGHS
Contracted: Leg extensions, 3sets...... 12-15 reps
Basic: Feet-crossed squats, 3 sets........ 5-7 reps

HAMSTRINGS
Contracted: Leg curls, 3 sets..... 10 reps

CALVES
Contracted: Standing Calf raises, 4 sets....... 15 reps

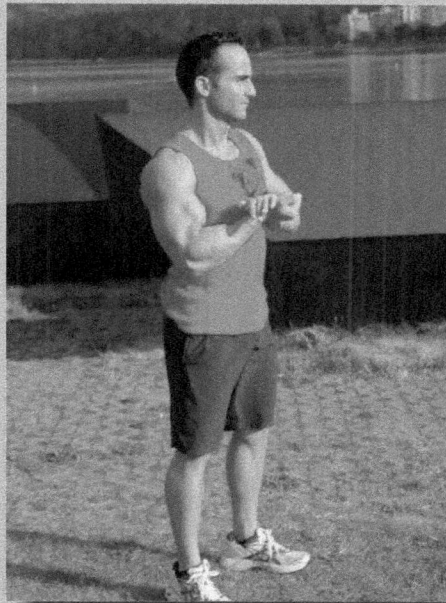

Day Two

SHOULDERS
Basic/stretch: Decline pushups (elbows out), 3 sets....... 12-15 reps
Basic/contracted: Upright rows, 3 sets...... 10-12 reps

TRAPS (NECK)
Contracted: Rear neck press, 3 sets...... 10-12 reps
Stretch/contracted: Side to side press, 3 sets...... 10 reps

BICEPS
Basic: Regular bicep curls, 4 sets..... 15 rep

TRICEPS
Basic: Forward tricep press, 3 sets...... 15 reps
Contracted: Tricep pressdown, 3 sets...... 15 reps

FOREARMS
Basic: Reverse curls, 3 sets........ 15 reps
Contracted: Reverse wrist curls, 3 sets........ 10 reps
Contracted: Palm up wrist curls 3 sets....... 10 reps

CALVES
Basic: Standing calf raises, 4 sets .... 20 reps

ABS
Basic: Reverse crunches, 3 sets .... 15-20 reps
Basic: Across the body crunches, 3 sets ....15 reps

CHAPTER 5

Day Three

CHEST
Basic/stretch: Incline pushups, 3 sets.......10-12 reps
Basic/stretch: Decline pushups, 3 sets.........
12-15 reps

BACK
Basic/stretch: Three chair dips, 3 sets ....
10-15 reps
Basic/stretch/contracted: Across the body
rows, 3 sets....... 10 reps

TRAPS
Contracted: Rear neck press, 3 sets........
12 reps

THIGHS
Contracted: Leg extensions, 3 sets....... 10 reps
Basic: Crossed feet squats, 3 sets....... 5-8 reps

HAMSTRINGS
Contracted: Leg curls, 4 sets........ 10 reps

CALVES
Contracted: Standing calf raises, 4 sets..........
15-18 reps

ABS
Basic: Reverse crunches, 4 sets........ 20 reps

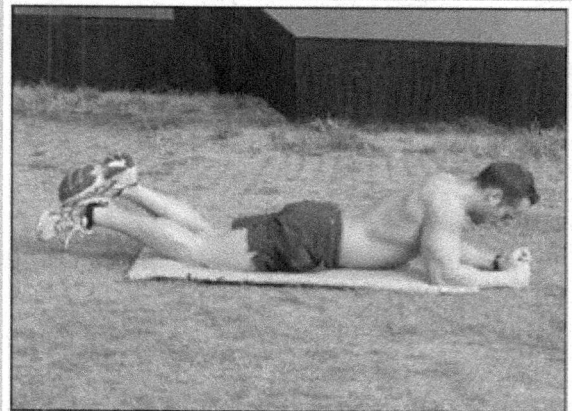

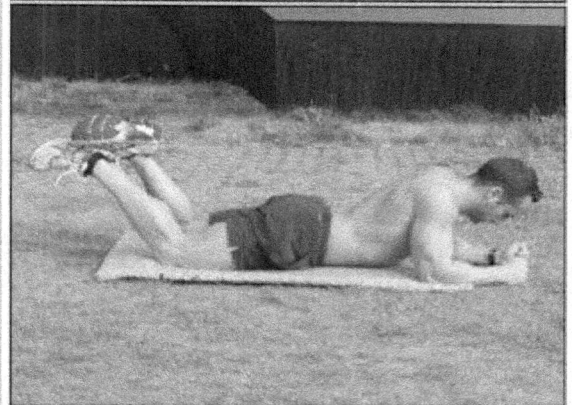

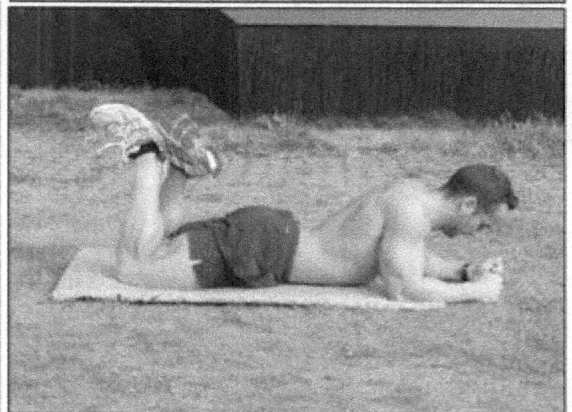

Day Four

CHEST
Decline pushups, 3 sets........ 15 reps
Incline pushups, 3 sets..........12-15 reps

SHOULDERS
Decline pushups (elbows out), 2 sets.....10 reps
Forward raises, 3 sets.........10 reps
Upright rows, 2 sets...........10 reps

CALVES
Standing calve raises, 3 sets.........20 reps

BICEPS
Regular curls, 3 sets.......12-15 reps

TRICEPS
Decline tricep extension or forward lateral press, 3 sets....... 7-12 reps
Tricep pressdowns, 3 sets.......15 reps

ABS
Reverse crunches, 4 sets.......15-20 reps

TRAPS
Rear neck press, 3 sets........15 reps

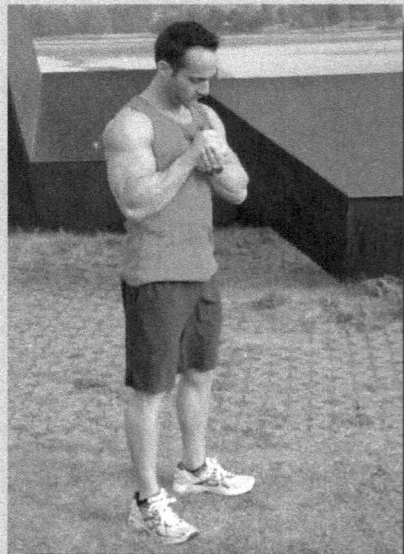

CHAPTER 5

Day Five

THIGHS
Leg extensions, 3 sets.........10-12 reps
Crossed feet squats, 3 sets.........5-7 reps

HAMSTRINGS
leg curls, 3 sets.......10 reps

CALVES
Standing Calf raises, 3 sets........10-15 reps

CHEST
Incline pushups, 3 sets.......10-15 reps

TRICEPS
Tricep pressdowns, 3 sets........10 reps
Decline tricep extensions, 3 sets.......7-9 reps

BICEPS
Regular curls, 2 sets.......20 reps

ABS
Reverse crunches, 3 sets.......15 reps

TRAPS
Rear press, 4 sets.......15 reps

CHAPTER 5

Day Six

CALVES
Standing calve raises, 3 sets.......18 reps

BACK
Thigh rows, 3 sets........ 10 reps
Across the body rows, 3 sets.....15 reps

CHEST
Decline pushups, 3 sets........15-18 reps

SHOULDERS
Decline pushups (elbows out), 3 sets........15 reps

THIGHS
Leg extensions, 3 sets.......10 reps

HAMSTRINGS
Leg curls, 3 sets........15 reps

ABS
Reverse crunches, 3 sets........20 reps

Perform this routine for 6 days straight resting the 7th day. This routine should be done for 3 weeks before moving onto Phase Two

Phase Two

* Remember with these exercises you perform the (Double-Impact) stress methed by performing a full rep followed by a half rep.

Phase Two
Day One

THIGHS
Basic: One legged squats, 3 sets.....7-9 reps
Contracted: Leg extensions, 2 sets.....10 reps

HAMSTRINGS
Contracted: Leg curls, 1 set..... 10 reps
*Leg curls, 2 sets......6 reps ....
Stretch/contracted: Stiff legged press, 3 sets.....10 reps

CALVES
Basic: Standing calf raises, 3 sets......15-20 reps
Stretch/contracted, 3 sets......20 reps

UPPER CHEST
*Decline pushups (elbows in), 3 sets......10 reps
Lower chest
Liederman press, 3 sets.......10 reps
Incline pushups, 3 sets.....10 reps

FOREARMS/BICEPS
*Reverse curls, 3 sets......10 reps
*Hammer curls, 3 sets......10 reps

ABS
Reverse crunches, 3 sets.......20 reps
Across the body crunches, 3 sets......15 reps

Day Two

UPPER BACK
Basic/contracted: Resisted pulldowns, 3 sets.....15 reps
Basic/contracted: Three chair dips, 2 sets..... 12-15 reps
Thigh rows, 2 sets.....10 reps

MID-BACK
Basic/stretch: Across the body rows, 3 sets.......10 reps

SHOULDERS
Basic: *Decline pushups (elbows out), 2 sets....10 reps
Stretch: Across the body lateral raises, 2 sets.....12 reps
Contracted: Forward raises, 2 sets...12 reps

UPPER TRAPS (NECK)
Basic: Rear neck press, 3 sets....10 reps
Stretch: Side to side press, 3 sets....10 reps

BICEPS
Basic: *Regular curls, 2 sets......10 reps
Contracted: *Concentration curls, 2 sets......10 reps
Basic: *Hammer curls, 2 sets.....10 reps

TRICEPS
Contracted: *Tricep pressdowns, 2 sets.....10 reps
Stretch: *Overhead tricep press, 2 sets....10 reps
Basic: *Forward lateral press, 2 sets.....10 reps

FOREARMS
Forearm press, 3 sets....10-15 reps
Palm up wrist curls, 2 sets.....10-15 reps
Palm down wrist curls, 2 sets....10-15 reps

Perform this routine alternating the days for 6 days a week for 3 weeks.

Phase Three

CHAPTER 6

*Perform exercises with a (Isometric pause) at the half way point of the exercise at the last rep for 20 seconds each on most self reistance exercises with an * mark next to them.

Phase Three
Day One

UPPER CHEST
Basic: Decline pushups (elbows in) , 3 sets.......15 reps

LOWER CHEST
Contracted: *Liederman press, 3 sets.......7 reps

UPPER TRAPS
Basic/stretch: *Side to side press, 3 sets.......7 reps

BICEPS
Basic: *Palm up bicep curl, 3 sets.......7 reps
Contracted: Concentration curl, 3 sets........7 reps

FOREARMS
Basic: *Reverse curl, 3 sets......7 reps
Contracted: Forearm press, 3 sets.......10 reps
Contracted: *Palm down wrist curl, 3 sets.......10 reps
Basic: *Hammer curls, 3 sets....10 reps

CALVES
Basic: Standing calf raises, 3 sets.......18-20 reps
Stretch: Slanted calf raises, 3 sets......20 reps

ABS
Reverse crunches, 4 sets......20 reps

CHAPTER 6

Phase Three
Day Two

UPPER TRAPS
Contracted: *Rear neck press, 3 sets......7-9 reps

SHOULDERS
Basic/stretch:: Decline pushup, 3 sets........15 reps
Contracted: Across the body pulls, 3 sets......

THIGHS
Contracted: *Leg extentions, 3 sets.....10 reps
Basic: One legged squats, 3 sets.......7-12 reps

HAMSTRINGS
Contracted: *Leg curls, 3 sets.....7-12 reps

CALVES
Basic/stretch/contracted: Standing calve raises, 3 sets....20 reps

UPPER BACK
Basic/stretch: Three chair dips, 3 sets.....12-15 reps
Basic/stretch/contracted: Across the body rows, 3 sets.....7-9 reps
Basic/contracted: *Resisted pulldowns, 3 sets......7-9 reps

TRICEPS
Contracted: *Tricep pressdown, 3 sets.....10-12 reps
Stretch: *Overhead tricep press, 3 sets......10-12 reps

Perform this routine alternating day one and day two throughout the week for 6 days straight for 3 weeks. Rest time between exercises 5 seconds.

Phase Four

CHAPTER 7

Perform a superset with a basic and contracted movement followed by an isometric (static hold) on the contracted movement for 20 seconds on the last rep.

Phase Four
Day One

CHEST (SUPER-SET STATIC CONTRACTION)
Decline pushups, 2 sets........12-15 reps........Liederman press, 2 sets........10 reps

UPPER BACK (SUPER-SET STATIC CONTRACTION)
Resisted pulldown, 2 sets.....10 reps.....Across the body rows, 2 sets.......10 reps

UPPER TRAPS (SUPER-SET STATIC CONTRACTION)
Side to side press, 2 sets....10 reps.....Rear neck press, 2 sets......10 reps

THIGHS (SUPER-SET STATIC CONTRACTION)
One legged squats, 2 sets......7-9 reps.......Leg extensions, 2 sets......10 reps

HAMSTRINGS
Leg curls, 3 sets.......12-15 reps (STATIC HOLD)

CALVES
Slanted calve raises, 3 sets......20-30 reps

SHOULDERS (SUPER-SET STATIC CONTRACTION)
shoulder press, 2 sets.....10 reps......Forward raises, 2 sets......7-9 reps

BICEPS (SUPER-SET STATIC CONTRACTION)
Bicep curls, 2 sets.......10 reps.......Concentration curls, 2 sets.......7-9 reps

TRICEPS (SUPER-SET STATIC CONTRACTION)
Forward lateral press, 2 sets........10 reps.......Tricep pressdown, 2 sets......7-9 reps

Reverse crunches, 3 sets......20 reps

Phase Four
Day Two

SHOULDERS (SUPER-SET STATIC CONTRACTION)
Across the body lateral raises, 2 sets......10 reps.....Resisted shoulder press, 2 sets.....7-9 reps
Resisted upright rows, 2 sets....10 reps.....Forward raises, 2 sets.....7-9 reps

CHEST(SUPER-SET STATIC CONTRACTION)
Incline pushups, 2 sets.......12-15 reps.......Liederman press, 2 sets......7-9 reps

UPPER BACK (SUPER-SET STATIC CONTRACTION)
Thigh rows, 2 sets.....10 reps......Siff arm pulldowns, 2 sets......7-9 reps
Across the body rows, 2 sets.....10 reps......Across the body rows, 2 sets ....7-9 reps

BICEPS/FOREARMS (SUPER-SET STATIC CONTRACTION)
Reverse curls, 2 sets.....10 reps......Hammer curls, 2 sets......7-9 reps

FOREAMS (SUPER-SET STATIC CONTRACTION)
Palm up wrist curls, 2 sets......10 reps.......Palm down wrist curls, 2 sets....10 reps

TRICEPS (SUPER-SET STATIC CONTRACTION)
Tricep pressdown, 2 sets....10 reps.....

LOWER BACK HAMSTRINGS
Stiff legged press, 2 sets......12 reps

THIGHS (SUPER-SET STATIC CONTRACTION)
Cross feet squats, 2 sets....10 reps.......Leg extensions, 2 sets.......7-9 reps

ABS
Across the body side crunches, 3 sets........20 reps
Reverse crunches, 3 sets.......20 reps

Perform this routine 6 days per week alternating the days for 3 weeks

Phase Five

CHAPTER 8

(Stretch-Pause-Training) Perform a 10 second pause on each rep on all pre-stretch movements.

Phase Five
Day One

THIGHS
Basic: Cross feet squats, 3 sets....15 reps
Basic: One legged squats, 3 sets......7-9 reps
Contracted: Leg extensions, 3 sets.....10 reps

HAMSTRINGS
Contracted: Leg curls, 3 sets........10 reps
Basic/Stretch: Stiff legged press, 3 sets.....5-7 reps (stretch pause)

CHEST
Contracted: Liederman press, 3 sets.....10 reps
Stretch: Decline pushups, 3 sets......5 reps (stretch pause)
Basic: Decline pushups, 3 sets......10-15 reps

UPPERBACK
Basic: Thigh rows, 3 sets......10 reps
Stretch/Basic: Three chair dips, 3 sets......5-7 reps (stretch pause)
Contracted/Basic: Across the body rows, 3 sets......10 reps

UPPER TRAPS
Stretch/Contracted: Side to side press, 3 sets.......5 reps (stretch pause)
Rear neck press, 3 sets.......10-15 reps

FOREARMS
Stretch/Contracted: Palm up wrist curls, 2 sets......5 reps (stretch pause)
Stretch/Contracted: Palm down wrist curl, 2 sets.....5 reps (stretch pause)
Basic: Hammer curls, 3 sets......10 reps

Phase Five
Day Two

SHOULDERS
Basic: Decline pushups, 3 sets......10-15 reps
Stretch: Across the body lateral raises, 3 sets......3-5 reps
Contracted: across the body pulls, 3 sets......10-15 reps

UPPER BACK
Contracted: Stiff arm pulldown, 3 sets......10 reps
Basic: Thigh rows, 3 sets......10 reps
Stretch: Three chair dips, 3 sets......5 reps

MIDBACK
Basic/Contracted: Reverse or regular upright rows, 3 sets....10 reps

CHEST
Contracted: Liederman press, 3 sets.......10 reps
Stretch: Decline pushups, 3 sets......3-5 reps

CALVES
Basic: Standing calve raises, 3 sets......15-20 reps

TRICEPS
Basic: Decline extensions, 3 sets.....5-9 reps
Stretch: Overhead tricep press, 3 sets.....5 reps
Basic: Forward lateral press, 3 sets......10 reps

BICEPS
Basic: Reverse curls, 3 sets.....10 reps
Basic: Hammer curls, 3 sets......10 reps
FOREARMS:
Reverse wrist curls, 3 sets....10 reps
Perform this routine for 6 days alternating days for 3 weeks.

Phase Six

CHAPTER 9

Phase Six

Perform the stress method (Ten by Ten) 10 full reps followed by 10 half reps to-wards the strongest muscle-building signal within the range of motion.

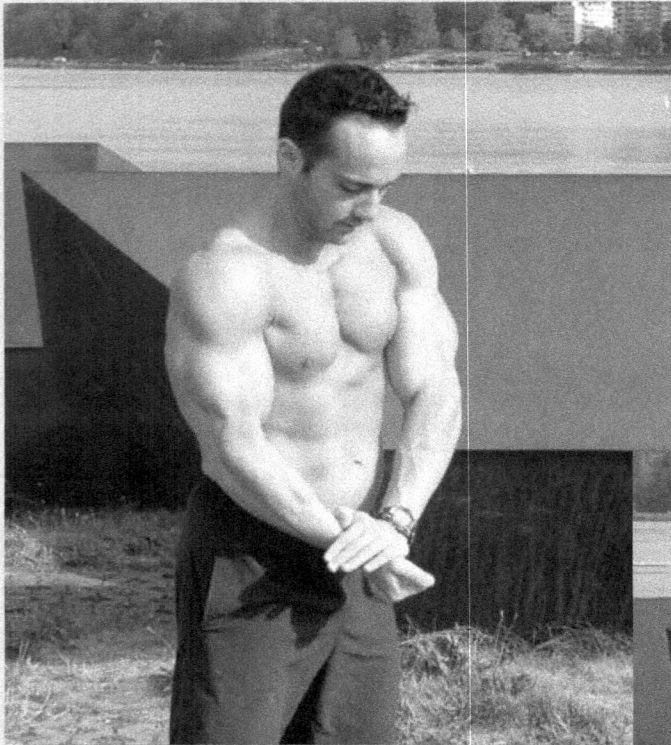

Start position

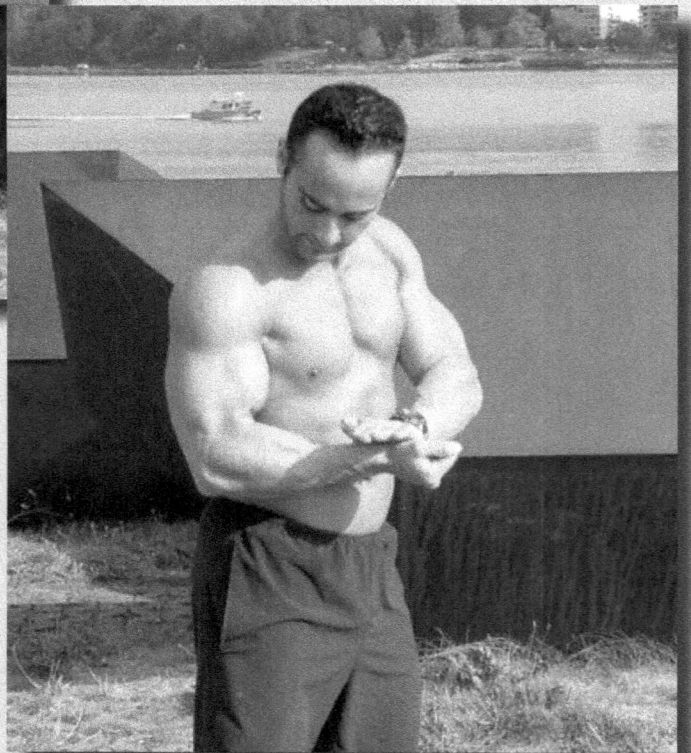

Mid-point

CHAPTER 9

Phase Six
Day One

(Ten by Ten) Stress Method

UPPER TRAPS
Contracted: Rear neck press, 3 sets.....9-15 reps

UPPER CHEST
Basic/Stretch: Decline pushups, 3 sets.....Ten by Ten

LOWER CHEST
Contracted: Liederman press, 3 sets....Ten by Ten

SHOULDERS
Basic: Decline pushups elbows out, 2 sets.....Ten by Ten
Contracted: Across the body pulls, 2 sets......12-15 reps
Basic/Contracted: Upright row, 2 sets......12-15 reps

BICEPS/FOREARMS
Basic: Palm up curls, 2 sets.....Ten by Ten
Basic: Reverse curls, 2 sets......Ten by Ten
Basic: Hammer curls, 2 sets....Ten by Ten
Contracted: Palm down wrist curls, 3 sets.....15 reps
Contracted: Palm up wrist curls, 3 sets.....15 reps

TRICEPS
Contracted: Tricep pressdown, 2 sets.....Ten by Ten
Stretch: Overhead tricep press, 2 sets....Ten by Ten
Basic: Decline tricep extension, 2 sets......10-12 reps

ABS
Basic: Reverse crunches, 3 sets.......20 reps
Basic: Across the body side crunches, 3 sets.....20 reps

Phase Six
Day Two

(Ten by Ten) Stress Method

UPPER TRAPS
Stretch: Side to side neck press, 3 sets.....15 reps

UPPER BACK
Basic: Thigh rows, 3 sets......10-15 reps
Basic/Stretch/Contracted: Across the body rows, 3 sets......10-15 reps
Basic: Three chair dip, 3 sets......Ten by Ten
Basic: Resisted pulldown 2 sets......Ten by Ten

MID BACK
Basic: Across the body pulls, 3 sets.....10-15 reps
Basic: Across the body rows 3 sets.....10-15 reps

THIGHS
Contracted: Leg extensions, 2 sets......Ten by Ten
Basic: Crossed feet squats, 2 sets.....Ten by Ten
Basic: One legged squats, 3 sets....Ten by Ten

HAMSTRINGS
Contracted: Leg curls, 2 sets.....Ten by Ten
Stretch: Stiff legged press, 3 sets........12-15 reps

CALVES
Stretch: Slanted calve raises, 3 sets......Ten by Ten
Contracted: Standing calve raises, 3 sets.....Ten by Ten

ABS
Basic: Reverse crunches, 3 sets........20 reps
Perform this routine alternating the days for 6 days straight for 3 weeks.

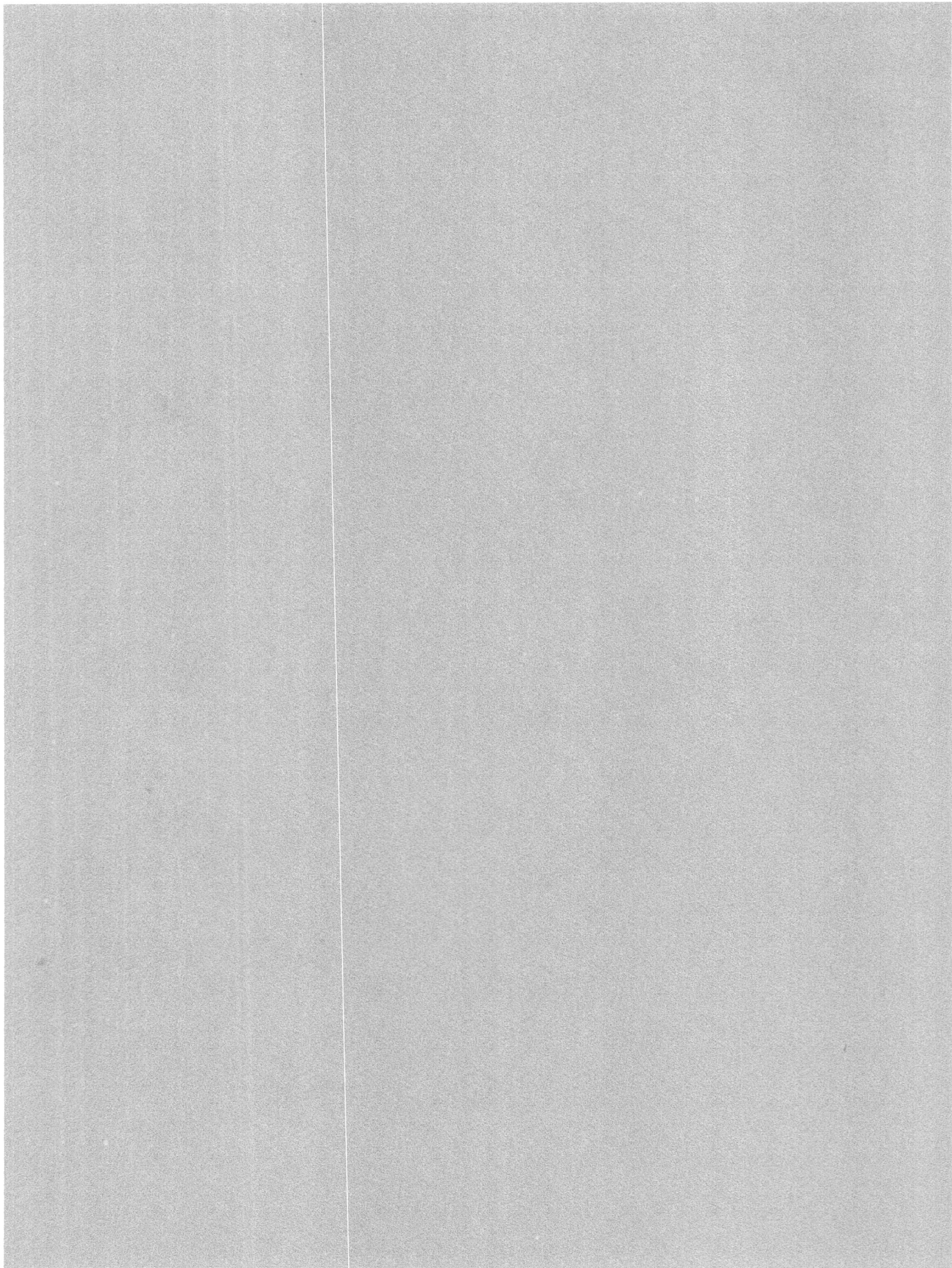

www.ingramcontent.com/pod-product-compliance
Lightning Source LLC
Chambersburg PA
CBHW081402270326
41930CB00015B/3389